MATT HOOVER'S
Guide to Life, Love, and Losing Weight

MATT HOOVER'S
Guide to Life, Love, and Losing Weight

By

MATT HOOVER

Winner of *The Biggest Loser Season 2* on NBC

and

SHERI R. COLBERG, PhD

Author of *The Diabetic Athlete, Diabetes-Free Kids, The 7 Step Diabetes Fitness Plan, 50 Secrets of the Longest Living People with Diabetes, The Science of Staying Young,* and *The Diabetic Athlete's Handbook*

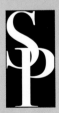

SKYHORSE PUBLISHING

Skyhorse Publishing books may be purchased in bulk at special discounts for sales promotion, corporate gifts, fund raising, or educational purposes. Special editions can also be created to specifications. For details, contact Special Sales Department, Skyhorse Publishing, 555 Eighth Avenue, Suite 903, New York, NY 10018 or info@skyhorsepublishing.com.

www.skyhorsepublishing.com

Library of Congress Cataloging-in-Publication Data
Hoover, Matt.
    Matt Hoover's guide to life, love, and losing weight / by Matt Hoover and Sheri R. Colberg.
        p.   cm.
    Includes bibliographical references.
    ISBN 978-1-60239-290-8 (pbk.: alk. paper)
    1. Weight loss. I. Colberg, Sheri, 1963- II. Biggest loser (Television program) III. Title.
RM222.2.H587 2008
613.2'5–dc22

                                    2008009753

10 9 8 7 6 5 4 3 2 1

Printed in China

Table of Contents

CHAPTER 1

Sometimes the Only Way to Go Is Up (and We Don't Mean Your Weight)

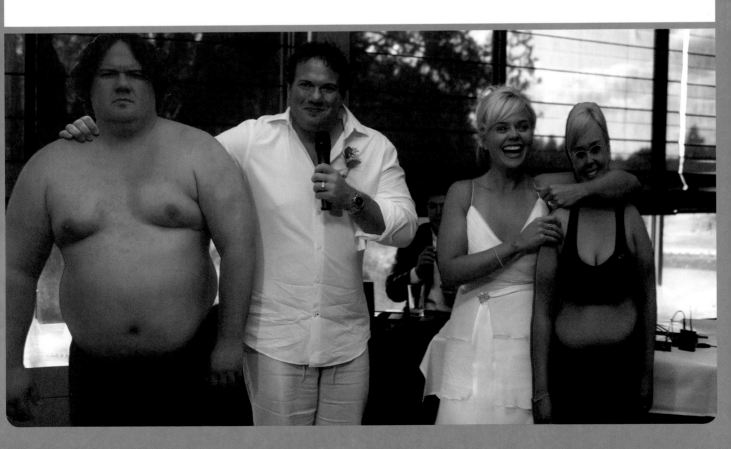

"Results not typical"

Don't you just hate to see those three words printed next to an impossibly skinny, fit person in form-fitting clothes featured in a weight-loss ad? Everywhere we look, we are inundated with images of beautiful people. It's what most of us strive to look like. We admire those people who just seem to have "it." They have the money, the fame, and the body. Did I mention the body?

Of course, results that you see in those ads just can't be typical, since no one is ever that successful at losing weight—or so I used to think. In fact, I never would have believed in a million years that I'd see the day when that message caption was stamped at the bottom of a picture of anyone I knew, let alone my own photo —but that actually happened to me just recently. Along with a bunch of other people that I actually know, my own "before" and "after" pictures are featured on NBC's *The Biggest Loser* Club Web site, and that pesky little saying is stamped right there at the bottom of all of them, mine included.

For those of you who may not know about *The Biggest Loser* TV show, I ask: where have you been? Seriously, though, that series is the only reality show to feature real-life contestants who have probably been called "loser" and worse at some point in their lives, all because of their body weight. While other shows feature people who want to be supermodels, B-list celebrities, tycoons-in-training, or even members of a deserving family seeing their wildest dreams come true, none carries the weight (figuratively and literally) of this widely popular show. It has to be the only show where the biggest "loser" is really just the opposite—an incredible winner.

The year I was on (2005), the show was in its second season. Fourteen contestants, most of us well over 100 pounds overweight, were selected to try to lose those excess pounds in what has got to be the most embarrassing way possible: under the close scrutiny of an unforgiving national TV audience. Given the unusual circumstances, you'd think we would've been put on some fad diet like Atkins or South Beach, since those are ones that everyone else tries these days. Instead, we were coached to use those tried-and-true, but not very popular, weight-loss "gimmicks" known as "diet and exercise." This strategy is a whole lot like the usual one that millions of Americans vow every New Year's Day to undertake, but the results on the show were hugely different for almost everyone involved.

In case you missed the finale of *The Biggest Loser 2*, I won. I lost 157 pounds, over 46 percent of my starting weight, during the show. As you can imagine, I was really proud of myself for what I accomplished in only nine months. Weight loss changed my life in so many incredible ways. I even met my wife, Suzy Preston Hoover (the second runner-up on the show), because of it. I can honestly say that nothing will ever be the same for me again, but the changes

in me and my life have definitely been all good—very good.

I'm writing this book to convince you that my results *can* be typical for every one of you, although I won't go as far as to guarantee that you'll end up with a new wife (or husband) from it! I won't hold anything back, though. By the end of the last chapter, you'll know everything that I learned from the doctors, dietitians, personal trainers, fitness consultants, and other weight-loss specialists hired by NBC to work with contestants on the show. I'm also going to share with you some of my own, previously unpublicized, secrets for taking a whole lot of weight off and keeping it off for good. With a little assistance from a really cool exercise physiologist and sports nutritionist that I know, Dr. Sheri Colberg, you'll walk away from reading this book with absolutely everything you need to be successful in changing your life for the better. For once, you'll be glad to say that you're a real "loser," too.

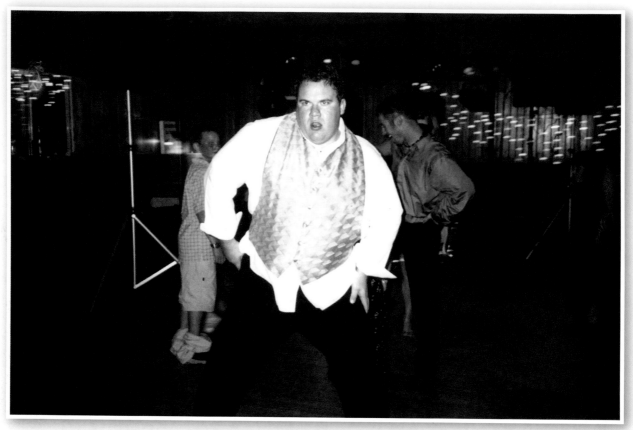

Showing off my dance skills at my best friend Richard's wedding.

On the Way Down

To start with, let me tell you a little more about myself and how I came to be a contestant on the show. As I'm sure you already know, I didn't get fat overnight, and I didn't get thin again that way either. But I definitely hit rock bottom before I got motivated enough to turn my life around, and I bet most of you will be able to relate to what I was thinking and feeling about myself at that point.

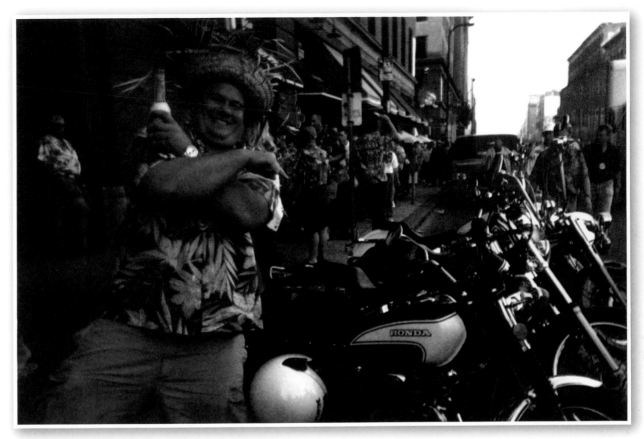

Pre-Jimmy Buffett party. Checkin' out the sweet "Hawgs."

I was born and raised in the small town of Belle Plaine, Iowa, in the heartland of America. I remember having a pretty happy childhood. I was a big boy—not much more overweight or obese than many of today's kids—and I did wear "husky" jeans.

Since I was a little overweight, my parents encouraged me to get involved in sports. I began wrestling in fifth grade and won my first state title that year, when I was the only 135-pound fifth grader in my weight bracket. From that time forward, wrestling

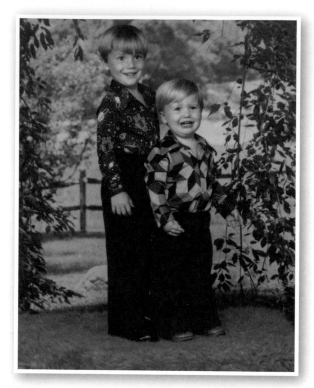

My little brother Timmy and I. Always a stylish guy!

My claim to fame as a teenager was becoming one of the best high school wrestlers in Iowa state history—by winning two state championships, earning all-American status three times, and representing the United States in the Junior World Championships. I was absolutely over the moon when Dan Gable, a former Olympic gold medalist and the University of Iowa wresting coach at the time, recruited me to wrestle for his team, which was the top college wrestling program in the nation. When I headed off to the University of Iowa in the fall of 1994, everyone, including myself, had high hopes for my collegiate wrestling career.

After my early successes in high school (or maybe because of them), I think my self-esteem took a real beating in college. Coach Gable and all of my teammates had high expectations for me, but although I was a member of the Iowa wrestling team for four years, wrestling in the 177- and 190-pound weight classes, I was never able to achieve any of my really important wrestling goals:

became my passion, and it helped me to slim down a lot in the years to follow. I didn't win very often when I first started, but with the support of my family and an excellent high school wrestling coach who saw some potential in me, I developed into a pretty good wrestler, if I do say so myself.

I never won an individual national title; I never competed on the international circuit when I was in college; and, most discouraging of all, I failed to make an Olympic wrestling team. I was plagued by injuries during my college years, but even realizing that didn't make me less disappointed in myself and my performance.

After my wrestling career ended in my early twenties, I really struggled with my failure to live up to the high athletic standards that had been set by and for me. I

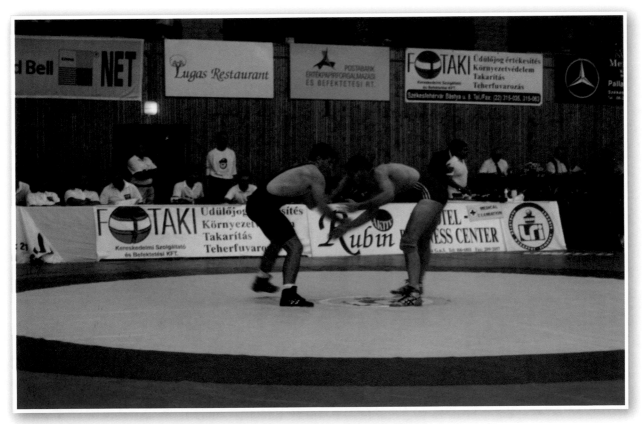

Representing the United States in the 1994 Jr. World Championships in Budapest, Hungary.

had come to identify myself as an athlete. If someone asked me to tell them who I was, I would say, "My name is Matt, and I am a wrestler." That was true, but the problems came later when I learned that I only knew myself as an athlete. Outside of that, I had no idea who I was. After my college career, I felt as if the true physical challenges in life—particularly related to my wrestling career—had passed me by and that I had failed miserably. I don't know if it was that overwhelming feeling of failure that led me down the wrong path or if it was that my whole identity was tied up in wrestling. Regardless of the cause, the result was that I totally lost the motivation to stay fit, healthy, and athletic, and my weight rose to over 340 pounds in a little over five years.

The Only Way to Go Was Up

How did I gain so much weight? Not long after college ended, I began drinking a lot, a whole lot. Don't get me wrong; I wasn't considered a loser at that point. Among my friends, I was usually the life of the party, and everyone liked to hang out with me. I think I used my sense of humor and partying to cover up the way I was really feeling. The fatter I got, the more I relied on making fun of myself for being "a big guy" before others could. It allowed me to put on a strong front, one that basically asserted, "I may be getting fat, but I don't mind. Look how happy I am."

I think most overweight guys do something similar. Rather than convey weakness and let others see that we may not be in control of our own lives, we try to come off as the jovial big guy. Although I had others fooled, I couldn't fool myself. I was hurting, and hurting right down to my core. No amount of alcohol or food could shrink the hurt. In fact, the more I tried to "medicate" away my feelings with both food and drink, the greater and greater the pain became. In retrospect, I now realize that the very method I was using to cope was bringing about my destruction, both physically and emotionally. I ended up developing serious eating and drinking problems; I became severely overweight and suffered in all aspects of my life.

When I surpassed 340 pounds at age twenty-eight, I still didn't consider myself a "fat guy" or a real loser, although I guess I should have. I think when my weight got that high, I had already sunk about as low as possible—there was probably nowhere to go but up. I had already given up on college, wrestling, and my first marriage, so what else could I possibly fail at? I had gotten married right out of college, but I doubt my first marriage failed just because I gained weight. I believe that it had everything to do with my behavior—the drinking and partying, the fear of failure and self-loathing, and the lack of motivation to do anything about any of it. I had a good job as a salesman, but I became so depressed after my wife and I split up that some days I would actually make my sales calls from bed while I ate leftover Chinese takeout. I can remember staying in bed for days at a time.

At my highest weight of 353 pounds, I always told myself I could change at any time. I let my hair grow long because I thought it made my face look thinner. I didn't tuck my shirt in because I thought it would hide that my belly was hanging over my pants. I kept the lights off in my house because then I wouldn't have to see myself in the mirror. In retrospect, I realize that I did these things and others to try and cover up the fact that I was a man with body image issues.

I tried to believe people when they said I carried my weight well. Check that—I did believe them. After all, I do have really broad shoulders. Only in the American Midwest can a guy be five foot ten, weigh over 340 pounds, and have people tell him he carries it well. (Hey, Sumo wrestlers carry their weight well, too, don't they?) My willingness to believe these comments is typical of how overweight people try to rationalize their weight gain, to excuse their excess weight, or to convince themselves that it's not really that bad or hurting them that much.

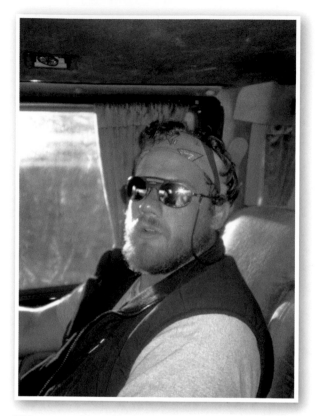
Whitewater rafting guide days in Colorado.

When I decided to try to get on *The Biggest Loser* TV show, I don't think that I was aware of how I looked. I remember lying on the couch watching the show with a cold beer in one hand while I munched down from an open bag of potato chips with my other hand. There I was, watching a bunch of fat people trying to exercise and lose weight. I saw them literally crying about how hard it was and thought to myself, "I wrestled at the University of Iowa for Dan Gable. I carried people on my back up the stairs of Carver Hawkeye Arena. There is nothing harder than that. I can't believe they are crying about that little workout they're doing. I should be on that show. I'd win!" Even in my totally unfit, overweight state, I had yet to truly accept that I was not in the same shape as when I was training and competing for Iowa's collegiate wrestling team.

As fate would have it, the following day I heard about a casting call for the next season of the show. It was being held just an hour and a half from my house in Iowa. Long story short, I went. Little did I know that that one impulsive decision, made on a whim, was destined to radically alter the course of my life. In February 2005, I was cast to be on NBC's *The Biggest Loser 2*, but I had no idea how much my life was about to change—forever, and definitely for the better.

My Promise to You

When it comes to weight loss, all "losers" are truly winners. Reality TV shows like *The Biggest Loser* may not actually seem very grounded in reality, but I promise that I can help make a "losing" outcome real for you. I will help motivate you to adopt better eating habits and a more active lifestyle that will help you lose all the weight that you want and keep it off for good. Whether you have ten pounds to lose or two hundred, I will share what I learned about fitness, dieting, health, life, and love on *The Biggest Loser 2* to energize all aspects of your life (yes, even your sex life) and help you achieve your goals—the end result will be a new and improved you.

Whether or not you've ever been an athlete is irrelevant. My results *can* be typical, and there's no reason why you can't experience the same success yourself—with a little guidance from me and Dr. Sheri Colberg. Read on, and make your weight-loss success worthy of a TV show.

CHAPTER 2

Being an Overweight Guy in Today's Culture Is the Pits

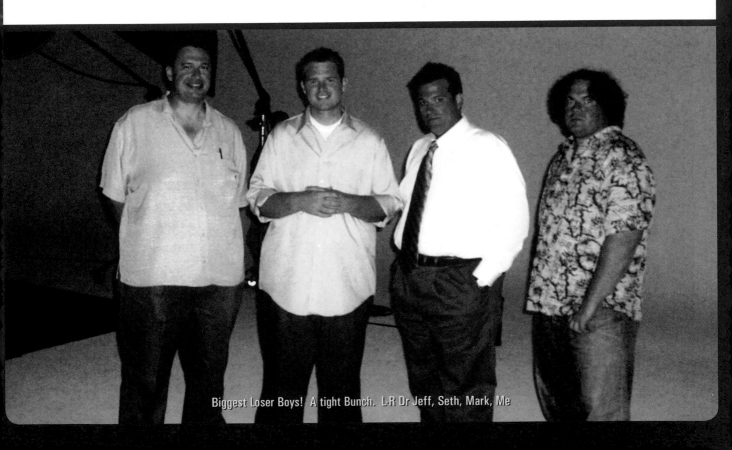

Biggest Loser Boys! A tight Bunch. L-R Dr Jeff, Seth, Mark, Me

You've all heard the saying, "If life is a bowl of cherries, how did I end up in the pits?" Let me tell you that becoming really overweight is one of the best ways to end up in Pit City. Think about it. Is there any aspect of your life that is unaffected by weight gain? You don't feel as well physically, your emotional health takes a nosedive, and your mind probably doesn't work as well either. I know that in today's culture, gaining too much weight wreaks havoc with your career, your social life, and your outlook on life in general.

When Your Body Image Takes a Nosedive

Only women have body image issues, right? *Wrong!* Men do, too, but admitting that seems to be the difference. On the whole, women are a lot more willing to own up to such issues. We live in a culture where first impressions are more often than not based on appearance. Guys, that means us,

too. Most of us feel that aging means that it's okay to carry around a spare tire. We look at young guys who are all buff and fit and think to ourselves, "Their time is coming; they can't keep that body forever." We would rather justify our body, or lack thereof, as an inevitable natural phenomenon.

When I was at my highest weight of 353 pounds, I always told myself I could change at any time, fooling myself with the long hair, untucked shirt, and darkened mirrors in my house. I played the role of the happy, fat drunk guy because it allowed me to cover up the *real* hurt that I had inside. It's amazing what we'll do to hide the fact that we have problems with our body image, isn't it?

Where did all this hurt come from? Let me go back to the beginning. When I decided to write this book, I experienced various emotions and thoughts. I wondered if anyone would want to read a book by someone who lacked professional training and whether I would be able to get all my thoughts on paper in a way that people could relate to. Perhaps the biggest question I had was, "What is going to make my story different than those in all the other weight-loss and self-help books out there?"

What I believe will make this book worth reading is the fact that it is *my* story, relayed to you with the honesty that I feel you

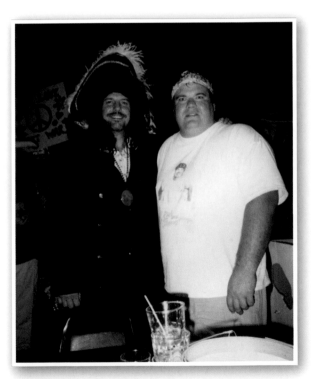

Doug Rassler (lead singer for the Cedar Island Band) and me. Yes, that is a picture of me on my own shirt.

deserve. I am not a doctor, a personal trainer, or a psychologist with years of professional training. I am a person who has fought the battle with obesity and will continue to fight it until my family has to send me off to the gates of heaven. When I worked hard to win the second season of *The Biggest Loser*—and simultaneously won back my health—I learned some life-changing lessons that I am happy to share with you.

The Beginning of My Downfall

Before I tell you more details about what happened on and after the show, let me describe a little more about what happened to get me to the point where I wanted to be on it in the first place. Believe me when I say that it didn't just happen overnight. As I mentioned, I grew up in a small town in Iowa called Belle Plaine, which was truly a great place to grow up. We could even leave the doors unlocked when we went on

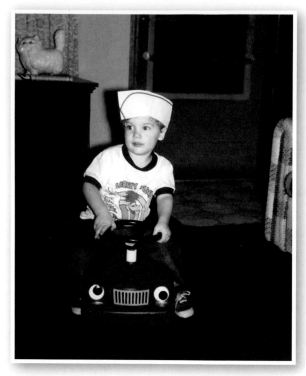

My first convertible! Traded it in for a Boxter almost thirty years later.

Although I became rather successful in wrestling, my introduction to the sport was a little rough. Unlike most fifth graders, I weighed 135 pounds. For those of you who are not familiar with the sport, in wrestling the idea is to compete against kids who are in the same weight class as you are. However, back then there weren't many fifth graders who were in my weight class.

When two of my classmates told me I should try wrestling, I quickly accepted their invitation. I went to practice and proceeded to take beating after beating from these two. At my first tournament, I was paired against my two practice partners, both of whom quickly smashed any hopes of a brilliant debut in my new sport by pinning me very quickly. I don't know why (maybe something was seriously wrong with me mentally), but I was hooked. Even after two good whippings on one Saturday morning, I could not wait to go to practice the next week and on to another tournament. The following week I was once again promptly pinned, but I was still

vacation, and my friends could come and go as they pleased in our house while we were gone without our having to worry.

Like in many small towns, in Iowa and elsewhere, sports were a big part of growing up. As I said, I began wrestling in fifth grade, which was actually a little late compared to the many kids who began in kindergarten.

undeterred. I wanted to be a wrestler. For the rest of the season, I was either pinned by everybody I wrestled, or I was the only kid in my weight class because there were not any kids big enough for me to wrestle.

I remember one conversation with my dad when I asked him if I could go to another tournament. I had yet to win a match in my new sport; when I had come home with a gold medal or trophy, it was because I was the only one in my weight class. The conversation went like this:

"Dad, can I go to the wrestling tournament this weekend?"

My dad replied, "Are you sure you want to go to another tournament?"

"Why wouldn't I?" That was the end of the conversation. After that day, my dad never questioned my desire again.

Even at a young age, I had the desire to compete. I didn't care if I won or lost; I just wanted to try and do my best. I finished my first year of wrestling without having won a single match. One of my proudest moments

that first year was when I went to a regional tournament in Minnesota. I was so excited because I was going to get to compete against kids from Minnesota, Wisconsin, Illinois, North Dakota, South Dakota, and Nebraska. I figured that even though I was probably the worst wrestler in my weight in Iowa, there had to be someone from one of those states that I could beat. I showed up, weighed in, and went to look at the brackets.

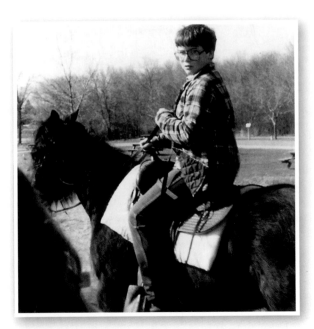

My pony, Babe. My mom and dad got her for me and she was my best friend when I was young. Sweet glasses!

I was the only kid in my weight class, which meant that I was a regional champ! I called my mom and told her I was the champion. I didn't have the heart to tell her it wasn't because I was the best wrestler in seven states; I was just the fattest. I'm pretty sure she knew why I had won, but she never let on.

I was lucky enough to have a great coach, named Al Billings, who somehow saw some talent in me and began working with me. Over the next couple of years, I actually started to win a few matches here and there and developed even more passion for wrestling. By the time I was in eighth grade, I was winning quite a bit. Wrestling had helped me to shed my baby fat, and the workouts had made me rather strong for my age. My freshman year, I played varsity football and also set a record for the most wins as a freshman on the varsity wrestling team. On the football field and on the wrestling mat, I was developing habits that would help me to excel at the varsity level. Off the field, though, I was developing bad habits that

would eventually destroy all of the good ones that I had been building.

One of the biggest complaints that I hear from kids when I travel to small towns to speak is that there is nothing to do. As a kid, I was no different. Since there was "nothing to do," I found something: I began drinking. My first taste of alcohol wasn't a good one. I remember gagging and trying not to spit it up. For some reason, I kept going and wound up drunk. I know I didn't feel too good the next day, but the first drink had been drunk, and I was pretty much hooked. People say alcohol is an acquired taste. I would have to agree. Although I didn't care for it at first, I grew to crave it.

In spite of the fact that our school had a good conduct policy, I spent my Friday nights during football season getting drunk after the game. It was common for kids to get busted and have to sit out games, but I never did. I didn't drink during wrestling season—until my senior year. Let's just say that going into my senior year, I may have developed something of a superiority complex. (Can any of you relate to this?) Here I was from little ol' Belle Plaine, yet every major wrestling school in the country wanted me to come wrestle for them. I didn't play football my senior year because of a back injury, so instead of playing football on Friday nights, I went on recruiting trips to various colleges around the country. I actually got alcohol poisoning on one trip and had a seizure at school the next Monday. Nobody said much about it, but I think everyone knew what had happened.

Nevertheless, I was beginning to feel invincible. I was drinking every weekend right up until the wrestling season started. I had made it all the way through high school without ever getting busted. The weekend before the season started, I went to a party. The party didn't get raided by the cops, but word got out. One night the superintendent's wife showed up at my house and told me that people knew and that I needed to do the right thing. Even though I had been denying

my actions up until that point, I called my coach and told him I had been drinking at the party. Coach said I had to go tell the principal, which I did. I was the captain of the wrestling team, and I had won a state title the year before without losing a single match … and I was about to miss out on the first five weeks of wrestling my senior year.

No miracle intervened and saved me. I sat out the five weeks. After that, I got ready to wrestle my first match of my senior year. I was chomping at the bit and ready to start

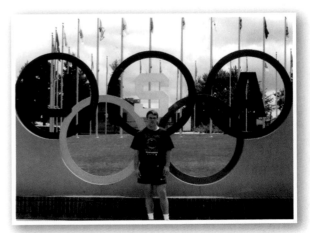

At the Olympic Training Center as part of the Jr. Olympic Developmental Camp, a camp designed to develop future Olympians.

down the road to my second state title. I hadn't lost in forty-two previous matches, so I assumed it would be business as usual. That night, though, when I was finally allowed to start wrestling again, I suffered my first loss in over a year. It was hard to take, but I came to learn that I had to get over it quickly in order to achieve my goals. I ended up winning the state title that year, but I missed out on being my school's all-time most winning wrestler by just a couple of matches, ones that, more than likely, I would have won if I hadn't had to sit out the first five weeks. After the season ended, it was back to the usual routine. During the week I worked out doing wrestling practice to prep for the University of Iowa's team, and Friday and Saturday nights I spent imbibing way too much alcohol.

A College Wrestling Career Gone Awry

I arrived at the University of Iowa as one of the top recruits in the country. I had turned down all of the other major wrestling schools in the country because I wanted to be a Hawkeye. In 1994, everyone wanted to be a member of the Hawkeye wrestling team. Iowa had been national champions several years in a row and Dan Gable was the head coach. If you went to Iowa to wrestle, you were pretty much guaranteed to be a national champ. At least that's what I thought. I had been a two-time state champ and a three-time Junior National All-American. The summer before I got to Iowa, I even represented the U.S.A. in the Junior World Championships in Hungary. I was good, and I knew it. After my first college workout, though, I found out that everybody else on the team was good, too. Nearly every guy in the room had been a state champ and high school all-American. My new workout partner at Iowa was an NCAA Division I National Champion named Joel Sharrat. After thoroughly beating me the entire practice, he leaned down close while I was lying on my back

"You're more likely to be discriminated against because of your body weight."

Fact. American society tends to reject obese individuals and subject them to severe stigmatization and discrimination in many social arenas, including education, employment, marriage, housing, and health care. If you're overweight, being treated this way may keep you from entering or succeeding in important and desirable roles in society, such as student, valued employee, or spouse. In short, discrimination can have a major, lifelong impact on you.

How you are treated depends on other factors, too. Body image largely reflects your culture, socioeconomic and marital status, life stage, and ethnicity; some cultures value bigger, rounder bodies. In the United States, the higher your socioeconomic status is, the thinner you're likely to be. What's more, married people weigh more than unmarried, parents weigh more than non-parents, and whites are less likely to be overweight (and more likely to value thinness) than Hispanics or African Americans.

and whispered, "Welcome to college." I had a lot of work ahead of me.

My high school coach, Al Billings, was one of the best high school coaches in the country. He guided me through my career like a drill sergeant, telling me when to run, what to eat, what techniques to use, and when to go to bed. In retrospect, I realize that his guidance was responsible for my becoming as successful as I had been.

Unfortunately, Coach Billings couldn't come with me to college.

I found out quickly that the coaches at the University of Iowa didn't care how good you were before you arrived. They were not going to tell you how or when to work out. Instead, they expected you to be an adult and figure out how to become a national champ on your own. I also learned that the professors didn't care if you came to class,

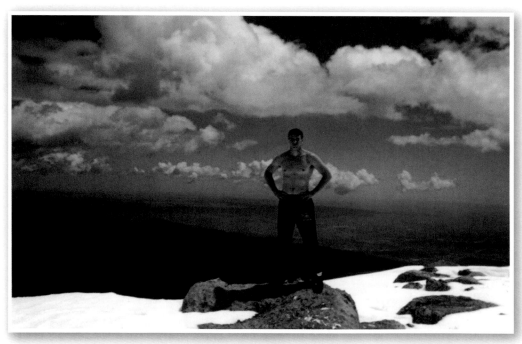

On top of Pikes Peak in Colorado after winning the Jr. World Team Trials. I felt like I was on top of the world!

and the bars around campus didn't mind taking your money. These factors were a train wreck waiting to happen as far as my wrestling career was concerned. I "redshirted" (sat out) my freshman year, but still managed to place second in both of the tournaments that I entered unattached that year. In one, I lost to Joel Sharrat, my workout partner, who was also a defending national champ, in the finals of the Northern Open at the University of Wisconsin; the other loss was to Lee Fullhart, a future national champ, at the Nebraska Omaha Open. I

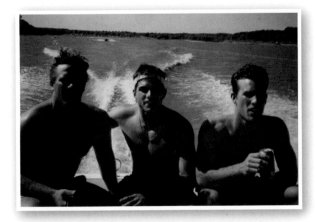

My good friends Joe Lotus and Steve Schroeder and me during college. Joe and Steve would one day become my agents. Who would have thought?

felt pretty good about my wrestling that year and believed that I was right on track for achieving my goals.

I lucked out with raw talent that first year. I learned a valuable lesson not long after: you can only get by on luck for so long before the guys who work hard catch up and eventually pass you by. My sophomore year I started getting hurt, and I couldn't figure out why. I had been relatively injury-free throughout high school and my "redshirt" year. The second year, however, I began to get injured on a regular basis. My grades suffered, and I eventually became academically ineligible to wrestle. I would work hard to regain my eligibility and then get hurt again; the cycle continued until I left school a couple of years later, only a few credit hours short of a degree.

After I left the University of Iowa, the rut I was in deepened and widened. I moved to Colorado, where I became a whitewater rafting guide. I fell in love with the water and the mountains. I began to meet people who were just like me: disenchanted with normal, mundane life and looking for excitement. I can't even begin to tell you how many times I heard someone say, "Yeah, man, I'm just going to take a semester off and do some traveling, you know, to see what's out there." I quickly became one of those guys. I saw some great places, but I never did get back to school to finish my degree.

Looking back now, it's a wonder I ever broke out of that cycle at all. I was a walking advertisement for how to become just like the people you hang around with. No matter where I went, I blended in like a chameleon. I learned that I never really had to be me as long as I was around others. I just had to be like them, and I would get along fine. I was a guide for a few summers before I decided it was time to go back into the real world and get my life together. I jumped around from job to job before I realized I wanted to wrestle again and finish my degree—but mostly wrestle.

I moved to Montana to attend Montana State University–Northern. They were NAIA national champs the year before, so I figured I would head out there and try to achieve what I couldn't at Iowa and win an individual national title. I was ineligible when I arrived, so I had to take classes and get nearly all A's in order to compete. I did that. I was in a "wrestle off" and won my spot. I was ranked third in the country in Division NAIA, and I hadn't even wrestled a match. The night before we were supposed to leave for the National Duals, my coach informed me that he had made an error in calculating what I needed to become eligible, and I was one credit short. You can probably guess where that oversight led: to hell in a hand basket in one quick moment. I never did compete in collegiate wrestling again, and I never bothered to finish my degree.

"The unhealthy practices that wrestlers often use to make their weight class before a competition, such as dehydration, have no lasting impact on long-term health."

Fiction. It is widely known that wrestlers, boxers, and other athletes who have to weigh in prior to competing to qualify for certain weight classes have traditionally engaged in unhealthy, short-term weight loss practices, like dehydration in a sauna, avoiding drinking fluids, and eating very little on the day of a weigh-in. The NCAA finally instituted some new rules about weigh-ins and changes in body fat percentages over the wrestling season that have helped reduce some of these practices and deterred some extreme weight loss behaviors.

Coaches and fellow wrestlers are primary influences on weight loss strategies. In a recent study, the primary methods of weight loss were gradual dieting (79 percent), increased exercise (75 percent), fasting (55 percent), sauna use to increase sweating (28 percent), and rubber/plastic

➡

suits (27 percent). Laxatives and vomiting are seldom used to lose weight nowadays, but some wrestlers still resort to such extremes.

What you may not know is that some of these common practices can have longer-lasting impacts on your health. In the past, athletes have lost their lives from taking extreme measures to lose drastic amounts of weight. It is unfortunate that such tragedies occurred, even more so because those incidents may have been avoided by using sound weight loss techniques. Wrestling-related incidences largely prompted the NCAA's changed policies, but these improvements have not necessarily made their way down to high school wrestling or up to international competitions, where extreme and rapid weight loss is still commonplace. Moreover, frequent, extreme weight cycling in high school wrestlers can delay growth and maturation and lead to future body image issues and eating disorders. Think twice about trying to lower your own body weight in any manner other than by minimally cutting back on calories (no more than 500 to 1,000 calories a day) and exercising moderately.

Gaining Weight and the Workplace Blues

I was in sales for quite some time. I would walk into a client's office and do a presentation and then walk out wondering why I didn't get a sale right on the spot. Deep down, I knew the answer. If I were a business owner, I would be leery of a sales guy who didn't care enough about his appearance to take care of himself. In sales, you can have all the knowledge in the world, but if you don't portray an image of self-confidence and enthusiasm, you won't get the account. A person's self-image will dictate how others see him (or her) as well. For me, being overweight and self-conscious made it nearly impossible to be an effective in-person sales rep.

Prior to going on *The Biggest Loser 2*, I worked for a company that produced segmental retaining walls. It was a good job that paid relatively well and allowed me to work from home, which was even better. We were the only producer of our particular brand in the state of Iowa, so my home state was my territory. I should have been able to set records for sales every year—I was the only guy selling my product in the entire state! I knew nearly everything there was to know about the retaining walls I sold. I could answer a question without even having to think about it or look it up. I worked with contractors, engineers, and private homeowners. Just about any person that wanted to use our block came through me in one way or another.

One of my responsibilities was to call on architects and engineers to get my product specified for use on various projects. This was the heart of the problem for me, and it didn't take me long to figure it out. There's just no getting around the fact that people base their initial opinion about others on appearance. You may already know this, but for me it was quite a shock. After all, I had a great product; my company had provided me with all the support and training I could ask for; I knew all of the technical specifications; and I could speak my clients' language and use their terms. How could they not want to buy from me?

Away from that career and looking back now, I think about what it would be like if I had been in the clients' shoes at that time. In my mind, the situation goes something like this.

On the phone: "Hi, this is Matt Hoover. I see your project is calling for segmental retaining block. I was wondering if I could have a moment of your time to tell you about my product and see if we can get it specified for your project. Can we set up a time for me to stop by and drop off some samples and tell you a little more?" (Pause for their response.) "Sure, tomorrow would be great."

On the phone, I always sounded very professional. I was respectful of the potential client's time and met my objective of scheduling a face-to-face meeting—so far, so good. Let's fast forward to the next day. When I arrive for the scheduled appointment, I'm running a couple of minutes late because I couldn't find the office. I can't remember the name of the person I talked to, but the receptionist knows who it is, so she saves me. I walk in the room to begin my presentation, and the person I am meeting looks a little uncertain. I proceed with my sales spiel, and the potential customer then says very tentatively, "Thanks. I'll see what we can do." I respond by thanking him for his time and telling him that I look forward to hearing from him. When I walk out of the office, thinking I got through it okay and hoping the sale comes through, I'm puzzled by why he looked a little surprised when I first walked into the room.

I'm not sure exactly when I stopped being puzzled, but at some point I finally figured it out. Imagine setting up an appointment over the phone with a very professional-sounding individual, only to have him show up late for a meeting looking like the proverbial train wreck. That is what I looked like. I came in with my shirt untucked, wearing pants that were

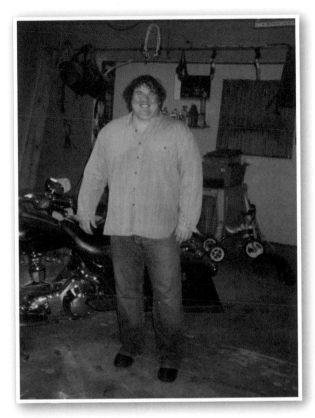
Hanging in my buddy's garage.

I told them that I would provide excellent customer service and take care of their needs when my appearance made it obvious that I couldn't even do that for myself. Like it or not, we are judged by our appearance. The way we take care of ourselves is apparent to those around us. People will treat us with respect, or lack thereof, accordingly.

My appearance wasn't the only thing that affected my job performance. My sheer laziness was the other. The problem wasn't that I worked from home; rather, it was that I was lazy *and* worked from home too much of the time. I was in such a deep depression that there were days when I could hardly bring myself to get out of bed. Thank God for cell phones: because of this technological marvel, I was able to make and return calls and still be somewhat productive without leaving my bed. I remember days spent hoping that no one would call that phone and then trying to decide if I should answer when it did ring. You should clue in that there is something seriously wrong with

saggy and baggy, with hair that looked like I had just rolled out of bed, and a beard that I wore because I was convinced it made my face look thinner. In other words, I was not very professional-looking. How could I expect the people to whom I was trying to sell my product to take me seriously when

"Even my doctor treats me differently because I'm overweight."

Fact. Unfortunately, studies have shown that even your health care providers (doctors, nurses, educators, and the like) are biased when it comes to your body weight. Although their prejudice may not be verbal in nature, the lack of response from professional and nonprofessional medical providers in responding to your needs as a bigger person (e.g., medical equipment, comfortable surroundings, properly fitting attire, etc.) is telling. In the past, studies have shown that physicians may view overweight patients as lacking in self-control, lazy, or sad. Despite laws designed to prevent discrimination based on appearance, unfavorable attitudes and practices among health care providers clearly persist when it comes to obesity, even to this day. Professionals whose careers emphasize research or the clinical management of obesity also show a very strong weight bias, and obese individuals—even if they work in health care themselves—are biased against others of the same size and weight!

you when you don't want to answer your business phone, especially when you know each call means a potential sale.

The thing about laziness is that being disorganized usually rides shotgun. I was the king of disarray. I can remember my boss asking me why I had receipts for gas in towns on opposite sides of the state on the same day. I would inevitably say that things needed to be taken care of and explain that, starting next week, I would be creating various territories around the state to eliminate the need to race all over putting out fires, so to speak. Being disorganized made my job more difficult and cost my company money. Rather than planning a schedule and sticking to it, I flew by the seat of my pants and ended up creating more work for myself.

A combination of laziness and disorganization must be to blame if people in sales aren't making ridiculous amounts of money. I know that was the case for me. Without a doubt, I know I could go back to that career now and double, or more than likely triple, my earnings. I am in no way saying that all obese people are lazy slobs, but I was. I'm sure there are more than a few people out there who wonder why they just can't seem to get it going professionally. I propose this theory: to get it going professionally, you have to get it going personally first. Take a long look at yourself to find the root of the problem.

From Former Athlete to Out-of-Shape "Loser"

There's no doubt that going from being a former college athlete to an out-of-shape one negatively impacts self-esteem. I wrestled at the best program in the country when I was in college. I worked out hard and often. When I dropped out of college, I felt like I deserved a break. I had put in a lot of years of workouts, and now it was my turn to be like everyone else. I went from one extreme to the next, and, for me, it was a rather smooth transition. I packed on my weight fast, and I packed it on good.

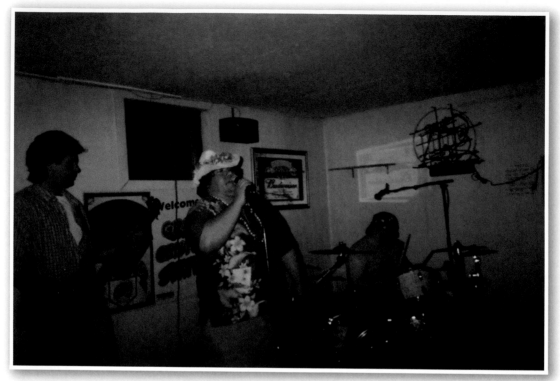

Singing some Jimmy Buffett at Grand Central Station.

I continually justified my weight gain as a temporary thing that I would and could remedy at the right time.

I think my extra weight affected me especially hard because I would always recall what good shape I used to be in. As my waist increased, my self-esteem decreased. I have met so many guys who tell me they are just like

I was—a good athlete in college or school—and now they are overweight. Here is what I think the problem is with guys like us. As athletes we have specific goals to achieve; we also have a coach in whom we put our trust to help us reach those goals. Fast forward: no sport or goals, no coach around to tell us what to do every day. Former athletes can

"Retiring from a successful athletic career damages almost everyone's body satisfaction and self-esteem."

Fact. A recent study looked at the psychological repercussions of transitioning out of an elite sport (in this case, they studied athletes from the Sydney Olympic Games in 2000) from a bodily point of view, hypothesizing that changing to a more sedentary state after retiring from competitive play would impact body satisfaction. They found this to be the case. Five months after retirement, former elite athletes had gained some weight, perceived their social value as diminished, and were substantially dissatisfied with their bodies, even if they continued to exercise (albeit at a lower training level).

Others have found that efforts made early in the athletes' careers to assist them in preparing for life after sports can certainly help. Finding a mentor to help you figure out where to go with your career after retirement and to offer guidance throughout your transition is critically important to your success in transitioning.

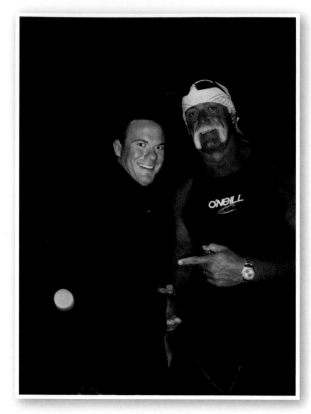

Hulk Hogan and me at the VH1 awards.

of us base our whole identity on one thing, such as our athletic achievements. When we no longer have that particular thing, whatever it may be, we fall apart. At some point, I ended up believing that because I didn't achieve my goals as a wrestler, I didn't deserve to achieve or be successful in anything else worthwhile in life. I held onto that belief until I went on the show and realized that I had more to offer in life, not only to others but to myself as well. Being a great athlete is awesome, but being a great person is even better (and longer lasting). Not reaching your goals as an athlete is no reason not to achieve them in the rest of your life.

Making a Career Out of Motivational Speaking

become like lost puppies. I have news for you: there is life after sports. There are goals to achieve besides athletic ones, and there are people who can act as coaches in other aspects of our lives if we just seek them out.

As I mentioned, when I was younger, I totally identified myself as an athlete. Many

I have to say that being on *The Biggest Loser* allowed me to experience some amazing things, but none has been as amazing as being given a platform to share my story and help others. Since my time on the show,

I have been traveling around the country, sharing my story and trying to motivate others to take their health into their own hands before it's too late. I love my new job, which still allows me to spend a lot of time with my family. I count myself very lucky to be in the position that I am in.

I feel that I have always been pretty good at motivating others. When I was a wrestling coach, I learned valuable skills on how to help athletes reach their potential. I implement many of the skills I learned back then now as a speaker. Essentially, I am still a coach; I just coach a different group.

I certainly didn't set out to be a speaker when I began the show. In my mind, a motivational speaker was a millionaire with walls and walls of diplomas, not a college dropout with weight issues. The first time I was asked to do an event, I was a little nervous. I wasn't sure what I was going to say, and before I went on stage, I realized that all I had to do was tell my story. I became less nervous because I knew that I couldn't mess up my own story. From that day on I was hooked, and I envisioned a lifetime of traveling around and helping to inspire others to lose weight and improve their lives. I hope that my message does inspire others to take control of their lives and their health.

My career enables me to constantly evaluate myself. I feel lucky to be in a position where I can step back and ask myself if I am living what I am teaching. If I ever get to the point where I don't believe the words that are coming out of my mouth, I will stop doing events. Being a speaker has helped me to step out of myself and take an objective look at my life now. I ask tough questions of myself and then answer honestly. One question that I ask on a regular basis is: If someone from the audience were to spend a week with you in your normal life, would they be able to see the principles you teach in action? I believe the answer is yes; however, that is not to say that I haven't struggled, and you'll hear more about those misadventures later on.

CHAPTER 3

You Are What You Eat (Literally)

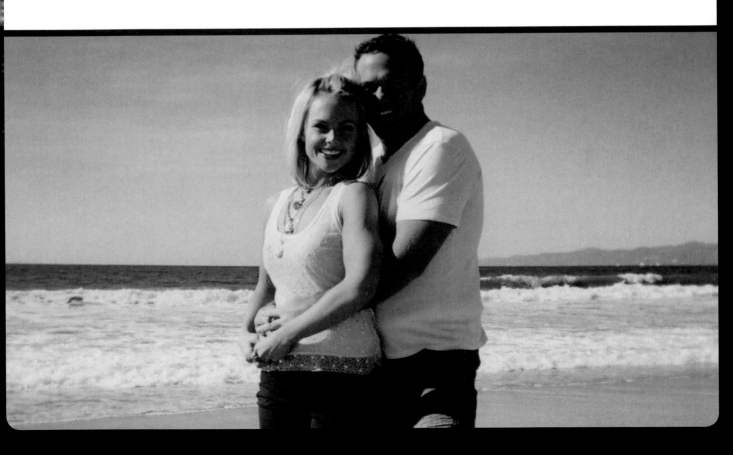

Ever since I was on *The Biggest Loser 2*, people have been asking me what my eating secrets are. I'd like to tell you that I came up with some undiscovered special food or foods that made the fat melt right off of me … but I can't. I did learn a lot more about nutrition and what I was eating, though, and I'm going to share that with you now so that you can improve your diet for the better, just like I did.

Leave the Fad Diets Behind

As soon as I got to the Biggest Loser Ranch, we all met individually with a dietitian. They didn't put us on any specific diet, though, and they certainly didn't recommend any fad diets like the Cabbage Soup Diet! Unfortunately, they didn't cook for us, so we had to do all of that ourselves. They basically taught us about the food groups—the basics like carbs, protein, and fat—and then let us figure out what to eat on our own.

Did you know that your body fat is made up of the same types of fats you eat?

When I was gaining weight, I never really thought about storing the same fat in my belly as was in my sixteen-ounce steaks. The main thing to remember is that gram for gram, fat has more calories, and there can be lots of hidden fat from butter, oils, and other stuff in your foods. Personally, I found it easiest to follow a higher-protein diet, avoiding most carbs, especially the refined ones, and I focused on eating more protein, vegetables, salads, and occasionally fruit. Staying away from a high fat intake also really helped me manage my calorie consumption better, and I think it was healthier for me.

My Typical Diet: Boring? Maybe, But It Works for Me

I think jocks (and former jocks) are probably some of the worst when it comes to spreading myths about food and exercise. How many of you have heard that you have to eat lots more protein to gain muscle?

"You can lose weight on any diet that is lower in calories."

Fact. The most popular diets recently focus on low-carb eating. But are they the best when it comes to losing weight? When it comes right down to it, the reason most diets work is because they're lower in calories. A recent study published in the *Journal of the American Medical Association* (JAMA), a respected scientific journal, compared the Atkins, Zone, Ornish, and LEARN diets to see if weight loss after twelve months in overweight and obese individuals—women in this case—differed. It turned out that they lost significant amounts of weight on all four diets by the end of the study year, but losses were greatest on the low-carb Atkins diet (almost twice as much as the other three diets, on average). Other studies have also shown greater weight loss with low-carb dieting, but only for the first six months, with no differences thereafter. Others have questioned the healthiness of such a high-fat diet, though.

Regardless of which diet you choose to follow, keep in mind that if you're eating fewer calories than your body

➡

needs, you will lose weight over the course of a year. As a general rule, you should be taking in at least 1,200 to 1,600 calories a day (probably the latter for most males) to make sure that your intake of nutrients is adequate and that you don't lose too much muscle mass.

Wrong! How about the one that says you can eat anything you want without gaining weight, as long as you work out? Wrong again! (It depends on what you eat and how much you exercise.)

I don't like to think too much about what I am going to eat, especially when I'm trying to lose weight or not gain any back, so instead I plan my meals ahead for every day of the week. This planning allows me to focus on other things I need to accomplish throughout the day and helps to curb cravings. I find that I give into cravings much easier when I am not sure what I am going to eat. At each meal I also drink a couple of glasses of water.

Breakfast. For years I didn't eat breakfast—what a mistake! Now, eating in the morning is simply habit. I usually eat two eggs and three egg whites scrambled and two pieces of sausage or a slice of turkey ham and drink a bottle of water.

Lunch. My lunch is nearly the same every day. I eat a bag of lettuce shreds, which are awesome because you can use the bag as a bowl if you are on the go. It's pre-washed as well, and the whole bag is around thirty calories. I put my dressing in a little snack-size baggie so I can squeeze it on my lettuce when I'm ready. (There is nothing worse than a soggy salad, which is what happens

Dr. Sheri's Tips on Which Popular Diets Work Best

Diet books are a dime a dozen, so how can you pick out which diet is right for you? Based on a recent analysis in *Consumer Reports*, some diets are definitely better than others when it comes to losing weight, even though almost all of them average around 1,500 calories per day. Here are Dr. Sheri's tips concerning the latest and greatest diet books and plans.

Eat, Drink, and Weigh Less: Written by a Harvard nutrition researcher, this book is scientifically accurate, but the diet, based on Mediterranean fare, has 1,910 calories, too many for most dieters to lose much weight, and there is little focus on exercise.

The Best Life Diet: Good discussions of and focus on exercise and emotional eating, but calories are not reduced until the second part of the diet, so initial weight loss is slow and potentially discouraging for many.

You: On a Diet: Lots of background info on appetite, metabolism, and behavior, but the diet itself lacks detail, is monotonous, ➡

and may be too restrictive for most; it starts with a two-week "rebooting program" to change behaviors first.

The Abs Diet: Now out in versions for both men and women, this diet focuses on eating six small meals a day; its extensive exercise program may be too difficult for beginners, and the emphasis on whey protein supplements is a turnoff for many.

The South Beach Diet: This diet is a slightly more permissive version of the Atkins version; it allows some fruits, high-fiber grains, and dark chocolate in the second phase despite being low-carb; its exercise section is lacking, though.

The Sonoma Diet: An updated, lower-carb diet with Mediterranean flair, this diet is healthy, but complex and needlessly restrictive; better exercise recommendations are needed.

Ultra-Metabolism: This diet includes an initial "detox" phase and a longer "rebalancing" phase to reduce toxicity, inflammation, and stress, but its premises go beyond scientific evidence; it's also considered overly restrictive and complicated.

The Low GI Diet Revolution: Based on the idea that lower glycemic index foods allow for greater weight loss, this diet promotes intake of all foods with a low GI and only some with a moderate rating; exercise is not well addressed, though.

Volumetrics: The diet aims to maximize the amount of food you can eat for a set number of calories, including broth-based soups, low-fat salads, and lots of veggies. This diet works, but still produces less than a 10 percent weight loss per year.

Weight Watchers: This diet emphasizes behavioral support (weekly meetings and weigh-ins) and scores high in long-term adherence (unlike some of the others); it has also been around for years and been effective for many individuals.

Jenny Craig: Individual counseling and meal plans are central in this diet, along with prepared foods; it has a high dropout rate, although people sticking with it can lose considerable amounts of weight.

Slim-Fast: This brand of controlled-calorie meal-replacement shakes meets nutritional and dietary guidelines, but has a high long-term dropout rate despite above-average short-term weight loss.

if you put the dressing on ahead of time.) On top of my salad, I usually put about four ounces of some type of meat, usually chicken, steak, or salmon. On days I don't feel like having a salad, I will eat a six-ounce steak, or I will fry some hamburger with onions, garlic, and a little cilantro.

Dinner. This meal always starts with a salad for me. When I am really hungry, it allows me to calm down and not feel like I have to devour an enormous quantity of food to satisfy myself. I like to pair a source of protein, such as steak, chicken, or fish, with steamed broccoli.

As I mentioned, I don't like to have to figure out what to eat, and I really don't like to spend a lot of time preparing it either, even though I often get my meals ready ahead of time. For instance, I make enough breakfast in advance for a couple of days and then just throw it in the microwave for a minute and thirty seconds. It makes for a fast, filling breakfast (and it saves on cleaning up pans and a lot of dishes every morning). The same

goes for meat for my other meals. I will grill a couple of days' worth of meals at a time and package them individually. Another reason I have my meals ready is so that I don't have a reason not to take my food with me and buy something less healthy to eat instead.

Good Carbs, Bad Carbs? But I Like Carbs!

Learning about carbohydrates is enough to make anyone's head spin these days. Are they good, or are they taboo? It doesn't seem like anyone knows for sure. Let me tell you what I do know, though: if you eat too much of anything, including healthy carbs, you'll get fat. When I do eat carbs, they come from low-cal, low-carb veggies like lettuce, other salad vegetables, broccoli, and the like. Occasionally, I'll eat a piece of fruit, but not too often. In looking back on how bad my diet was before I went on the show, I realized that for my health, I just had to cut certain things out of my

"It's possible to lose eight or more pounds in just a week of dieting."

Fact. While you can lose that amount of weight or more in a week, there are two things that you should realize. First, in the first week of a diet, most of the weight you lose is truly from water losses. Your body stores extra water with carbohydrates in muscle (glycogen), and when you're restricting your calorie intake, you'll lose the glycogen and the water stored with it. You haven't lost much fat that first week, though, since fat typically contains about 3,500 calories per pound. When and if you start eating and drinking more normally again, that weight is likely to come right back on. Second, the longer you've been on a diet, the harder it becomes to lose weight quickly, for a variety of reasons, including the fact that later losses come more from fat (which is more calorie dense per pound) and less from water.

diet completely—particularly things that are easy to eat way too much of and that are packed with calories, like potato chips, snack crackers, cookies, and other highly processed foods made with white flour and white sugar. My general rule now is not to buy them, and then I'm a lot less likely to ever eat them. If I do have some, I put a reasonable serving in a small bowl and put the rest of the bag away before I begin eating. I've actually found that other foods are a lot more filling (like chicken or fish with salad), so I figure I'm better off eating those foods for a lot of different reasons. Anything

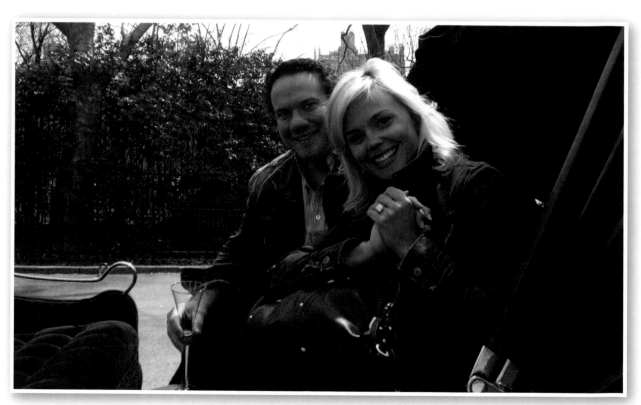

Suzy and I in Central Park, New York, shortly after we got engaged live on The TODAY Show.

"Your weight loss while you're dieting is likely to be consistent and continual."

Fiction. As mentioned, it's easy to lose weight quickly during the first week or two of a diet. After that, you start losing more fat, and fat stores are calorie-dense. A pound of muscle only contains about 2,000 calories, but a similar weight of fat stores contains almost twice that, or 3,500 calories. Thus, weight loss that comes mainly from fat stores is slower. Also, the energy expenditure from your body's basal needs and any physical activity you do during each day goes down as you lose weight. It takes more energy to move a heavier mass, and the more weight you lose, the less energy you burn getting from point A to point B. It also takes less energy to maintain a body that is a smaller size, so even your resting energy needs go down. For all of these reasons, most people hit a plateau in their weight loss somewhere along the way, and you probably will too, unless you either add more movement into your day or cut back the calories some more. Don't cut back too far, though, or you'll likely

➡

> end up putting your body into "starvation mode," which will make it more energy efficient and less likely to lose weight easily.

with fiber is a lot more filling, and the proteins stick with you a long time, too. Things with a lot of fat and calories, like candy bars, are just not nearly as filling for as long.

Matt and Suzy's Favorite Eats

Anyone can lose weight on a diet, and some diets may make you lose more than others in the short-term, but in the long run, none of them is any good for losing weight and keeping it off. You should avoid some foods and diets altogether, particularly ones that are likely to unbalance your metabolism. When it comes to eating, some people don't have the luxury of being able to eat anything they want. My wife and I are two of those people. If I don't keep my eating clean, so to speak, I can gain ten pounds in one week. If you are lucky enough to have a great partner in your life with similar goals and aspirations, it shouldn't be too hard to get her (or him) on the same page when it comes to nutrition. Eating right becomes much easier when the people who live in your house or are a part of your life are willing to do it with you.

Suzy and I like different things, but in order to help each other, we try to eat the same types of foods. The key to any diet, especially when it's your eating plan for the rest of your life, is to eat and prepare foods you enjoy. By making foods that you like, you will be able to move away from saying you are dieting (if you are) and instead say that you're just eating sensibly.

We eat a variety of foods and prepare them in different ways. One of our favorite things to prepare is spaghetti squash. A lot of people don't even know what spaghetti squash is, even though they have probably walked by it in the grocery store a hundred times. This particular squash is a sort of football-shaped yellow vegetable with a very hard outer skin. We prepare it by cutting it in half and covering it with saran wrap. We microwave it for seven to nine minutes; when it is done, we take a fork and scrape it out. Amazingly, once it's out of the squash shell, it looks just like spaghetti (hence the name). The great thing about this vegetable is that it's versatile. We have eaten it with meat sauce like real spaghetti, minus the pasta carbs, as well as just plain. It has a nice little crunch when prepared properly, unlike other types of squash, which become mushy.

Asparagus is also one of our favorite vegetables. It can be prepared in so many different ways, and each way gives it a different flavor. We have baked it, fried it, grilled it, and even had it raw in salads. Asparagus, like most other green vegetables, is packed with vitamins and nutrients. One side note: expect to have a strong odor to your urine after eating it; I'm not sure why that is, but it is nothing to be alarmed about.

Broccoli is also a staple in our refrigerator. It is low in calories and can really fill you up. You can eat a ton of broccoli without having to think about calories. We spray a little I Can't Believe It's Not Butter! on it, sprinkle with a little parmesan cheese, and eat it as a snack between meals as well.

Almost every grocery store now carries shredded lettuce in bags. We love those little bags. They make great lunches as well as snacks. Try to pick the ones that have darker green lettuce, which is packed full of fiber, vitamins, minerals, iron, and calcium,

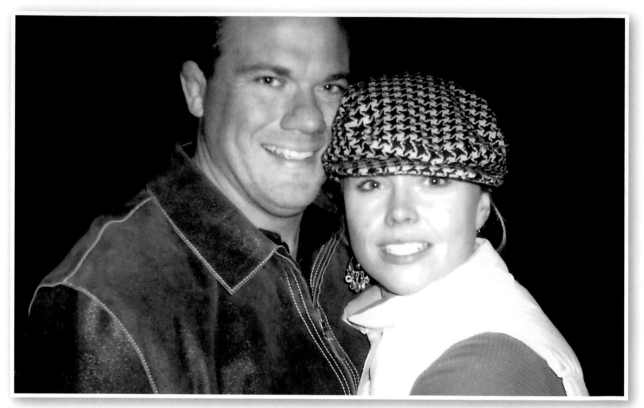

Late night in Las Vegas.

instead of the colorless iceberg lettuce that is almost devoid of extra nutrients. When we are on the go, we can put a little dressing and some protein right in the bag with it and eat it straight. We have lots of chicken in our freezer that we can easily add to complete it. Chicken is low in fat and high in protein and is another food that can be prepared in many different ways. I like to cook up several pieces and eat them during the week for lunch.

I grew up in a state that produces some of the best steaks in the country, so it is little wonder that I love eating beef. I grill everything from hamburgers to steak. Today,

"You're only overweight because you have no willpower when it comes to eating."

Fiction. Your body weight is determined by a large number of factors, including your genes (affecting your body's ability to burn calories and store fat), level of physical activity, diet, cultural attitudes, and financial situation. Apparently, your brain and fat cells also have something to say about what and when you eat, so you can't blame all of your weight gain on your lack of willpower, your environment, or your genes.

In fact, a new study recently showed that an urge to snack, even after just eating, may be due to an overactive chemical feedback system that regulates your appetite, food intake, fat metabolism, and body weight together. Remember the "munchies" that people get when they're exposed to the cannabinoids in marijuana? Well, there's an endocannabinoid (EC) system in your brain, and when it's activated, it increases your drive to eat and decreases your ability to feel satisfied. In fact, there are cannabinoid receptors all over your body, including in your brain, fat cells, stomach, and intestinal tract. The EC system interacts with other hormones to make you feel hungrier and increase your body fat stores. It has also been shown to be overactive in obese individuals. Other hormones like leptin and insulin also interact with the EC system, telling the brain how much you have eaten and how much fat has been stored.

Knowing that you have the EC system working against you makes a stronger case for avoiding certain types of foods: it appears that high-fat, high-carbohydrate foods are more likely to activate it and drive you to eat even more. You can also trick the system using some proven strategies that help you defuse the urge to snack or overeat, such as waiting five to fifteen minutes for a craving to pass, distracting yourself with other activities (such as taking a walk), or even drinking a glass of water or other calorie-free fluid. Also, choose foods that increase your sense of fullness (ones high in water and fiber content), such as fruits and vegetables. Finally, realize that it takes about twenty minutes for your brain to receive the message from your stomach that it's full, so slow down when you eat to promote earlier feelings of satiety.

At present, one weight loss drug called Rimonabant is actually available to block EC receptors. Although it doesn't appear to cause more than moderate weight loss in users, even their 5 percent weight loss, on average, after a year greatly reduced their risk for health problems like type 2 diabetes and cardiovascular disease.

The NWCR: What Works Best over the Long Haul for Maintaining Weight Loss

Not surprisingly, 98 percent of the members of the National Weight Control Registry (NWCR, found online at www.nwcr.ws), who each lost at least thirty pounds and kept it off for a year minimum to qualify, report having modified their intake in some way to lose weight. However, only a minority of them (17 percent) currently consume a low-carbohydrate diet to keep their weight controlled, regardless of what diet they followed to lose the extra pounds. On average in their diets, about 50 percent of their calories are carbo- hydrates, 30 percent are fat, and the remainder (about 20 percent) ➡

is protein—no lifelong Atkins or South Beach diet for them! By way of comparison, current dietary guidelines recommend intakes in the range of 45 to 65 percent of calories from carbs, 20 to 35 percent from fat, and 10 to 35 percent from protein sources.

The individuals who regained the most weight had higher calorie intakes, ate more fast foods and fat, and had lower levels of physical activity, whereas those who maintained their weight loss continued to consume a lower-calorie diet with moderate fat intake, limited fast food, and exercised a lot. Another key point is that the dietary selections of the successful losers are limited, meaning that they have less variety in their diets within all food groups. Other investigators have shown that when people are given many food choices (such as at buffet restaurants), they eat more, so there may be something to keeping fewer varieties of foods around, particularly the less healthy ones, when it comes to losing weight *and* keeping it off.

quality beef can be nearly as lean as chicken and is also a great source of protein. Grilling is an excellent way to prepare all types of meat. We try to minimize frying because the oil adds lots of calories; generally we prefer to grill or bake our meat instead.

As for other protein sources, Suzy and I are both fans of fish. She likes to eat salmon, which is high in healthy omega-3 fats. She wraps it in foil and cooks it either in the oven or on the grill. I love white fish, such as halibut or cod. We do occasionally lightly fry these types of fish up in a nonstick pan with a little bit of olive oil, which adds a few calories, but at least they're really healthy ones.

Every now and then, almost everyone craves some sort of sweets. You can definitely add both of us to that list. Nowadays, rather than baking cookies, we tend to enjoy some things that are sweet, but lower in calories. Sugar-free pudding and gelatins are probably the most common things that we reach for when we have a craving, and either one can be jazzed up with a little fat-free whipped cream. There are so many flavors that it is hard not to find something you like. We usually make up gelatin in advance and store it in the refrigerator, but the great thing about pudding is that it can be prepared quickly in case of an emergency craving.

When it comes right down to it, we like lean meats and fresh veggies. We don't buy a lot of frozen vegetables—not because they aren't as good for you, but rather because buying fresh helps us make sure that we eat the vegetables in our fridge. They are more expensive, and we don't want to waste our money by letting them go to waste. We also like to have a variety of foods. My general rule is that if it comes from the ground (like veggies or fruits) or eats what comes from the ground and is in its natural state, it is probably not too bad for your health. If it comes from a bag in the potato chip or cookie aisle, though, stay away from it!

Take It from Me: There's a Right and a Wrong Way to Eat

I'm just a regular guy, and I still want to load up on three platefuls of food when I go to a buffet. The difference now, though, is that I choose not to eat that much. Here's a quote I like: "Nothing tastes as good as being thin feels." I've learned that not skipping breakfast and eating balanced meals throughout the day actually keeps me from getting too hungry. Don't get me wrong; I still get cravings and want to go to those all-you-can-stuff-yourself-with-and-still-walk places, but I know that to keep my weight in check I really have to avoid them. It's all about portion control and reasonable eating.

Here's a sample menu for my week these days:

Monday. For breakfast, I have two eggs, three egg whites, and two sausage patties. Lunch consists of one bag of lettuce shreds, three tablespoons of sesame dressing, and four ounces of sliced, grilled chicken. My dinner is a green salad with dressing, followed by a stir-fry dish with vegetables, chicken, and steak.

Tuesday. Now here's some variety: with my breakfast of eggs and egg whites, I have three ounces of turkey ham instead of sausage patties. Lunch is a salad with dijonaise dressing instead of sesame, along with one and a half grilled salmon patties. My dinner

salad tonight comes with a six-ounce steak and steamed broccoli (as much as I care to eat).

Wednesday. I eat the same breakfast as Monday, but for lunch, I have eight ounces of lean hamburger cooked in a pan with chopped onions, pickles, fresh garlic, and cilantro. On top, I put about three tablespoons of ketchup and mustard. My dinner consists of a green salad with dressing, six ounces of grilled chicken breast, and asparagus (one of my favorite veggies).

Thursday. I repeat my Tuesday breakfast (I typically alternate days during the week), and then for lunch I have salad with sesame dressing, along with four ounces of grilled and sliced steak. After a dinner salad later, the rest of my meal is made up of six ounces of cod spritzed with I Can't Believe It's Not Butter! spray and sprinkled with celery salt (lightly!), as well as zucchini sprayed with the same and sprinkled with parmesan cheese.

Friday. I eat the same breakfast as Monday and Wednesday and opt for the lettuce

"All weight-loss diets are equal when it comes to being heart-healthy and preventing type 2 diabetes."

Fiction. When it comes to diabetes prevention and a healthy heart, diets can have differing effects. Normally, a diet low in saturated fats and rich in whole grains, vegetables, and fruit is recommended for reducing the risk of obesity, cardiovascular disease, and type 2 diabetes. Given the widespread interest in high-fat (Atkins diet) and high-protein (Zone diet) diet alternatives, a recent study in *Diabetologia* examined their effects to find out which is best. The results are interesting. In the overweight women with pre-diabetes (insulin resistance) who were studied for a year, a lower-carb, higher-protein diet like the Zone diet (comprised of 40 percent of calories from carbs, 30 from protein, and the last 30 from fat) may be the most appropriate for reducing the risk of heart disease and type 2 diabetes.

If you follow a higher-carb diet, you may do okay, but only if you pay careful attention to the types of carbs you eat and increase your intake of high fiber whole grains,

➡

legumes (beans), vegetables, and fruits, while cutting back dramatically on your intake of refined sugars and carbs (e.g., regular sodas, white flour products, white sugar, white rice, and white potatoes) and saturated fats. If you follow a high-fat diet like Atkins, you'll likely lose weight in the short run, but your cholesterol levels (and other blood fats) can go up too high if you stay on the diet over the long haul.

Dr. Sheri's Dietary Tips for Good Health and Longevity

- **Improve the heart-healthiness of your diet.** As far as your health goes, you really can't go wrong with a diet containing fish, veggies, fruits, whole grains, some olive oil, and limited amounts of red wine and dark chocolate.
- **Consume at least three to five vegetables and two to three fruits a day.** For optimal health, choose colorful fresh or frozen produce, and eat whole fruits rather than drinking juices,

which lack fiber. All of these plant foods are chock full of vitamins, minerals, and antioxidant-rich phytonutrients.

- **Eat more fiber-rich foods.** Fiber lowers blood sugar levels and cholesterol and is found in dried beans, whole grains, bran, veggies, fruit, and nuts. Men need at least thirty eight grams per day, and women should eat twenty five or more to promote regularity and overall health.

- **Eat fish two to four times per week.** An increased intake of essential omega-3 fats (found in cold-water fish like salmon, mackerel, and herring) boosts heart health and lowers your risk of many other health problems, including memory loss and dementia as you age.

- **Drink plenty of liquids.** Drink at least four to six glasses of liquid each day—preferably water or other non-caffeinated, non-caloric drinks—and eat more foods with higher water contents like melons and many vegetables. Drinking a glass of water before meals is a great way to fill up your stomach to keep yourself from overeating.

- **Eat more live-culture yogurt.** The probiotic effect of yogurt may improve your health by preventing illness and ➡

limiting inflammation. Go for the lower-fat varieties, and get the sugar-free ones to reduce your calorie and refined sugar intake.

- **Drink alcohol moderately.** Consuming one (for women) to two (for men) alcoholic drinks per day may be beneficial, but don't drink more than that. Keep in mind that drinking in moderation (as opposed to in excess) is not only critical in terms of your heart health and cancer risk, but also in keeping your calorie intake in check.

- **Spice up your foods.** Using spices found in onions, turmeric, black pepper, cinnamon, ginger, thyme, cumin, oregano, basil, sage, curry, and garlic may benefit your health in a variety of ways. Adding spices also jazzes up your meals and makes them more appealing.

with dijonaise dressing at lunch, with four ounces of chicken breast. For dinner, I enjoy a salad with dressing, steak, and broccoli.

Saturday. I eat an alternate breakfast on Saturdays, which consists of two eggs, three egg whites, and four slices of turkey bacon (it has less fat than the regular type). For lunch, I go wild and have a broccoli salad with grilled chicken, followed by a dinner of six ounces of grilled chicken and spaghetti squash made with garlic, Laughing Cow cheese, and butter spray.

Sunday. This is the day I eat green peppers, onions, sausage, ham, and some cheese cooked in with my usual eggs and egg whites for breakfast. My wife and I usually go out to lunch, but I try to eat responsibly. For dinner, I'm back to a salad with dressing, along with some lasagna made with sliced zucchini in place of the traditional pasta noodles.

I realize that mine is a pretty mundane menu, but it is truly typical of what I eat.

By switching salad dressing and meats, it doesn't seem like I am eating the same foods every day, and I haven't gotten bored with them yet. I have to admit that every couple of weeks, I will go to Baskin Robbins and have two scoops of chocolate peanut butter ice cream in a dish. An occasional treat is good for the soul, I think, as long as you have it in moderation. The real trick is to eat it slowly and savor every bite!

CHAPTER 4

Close Your Mouth and Move Your Feet

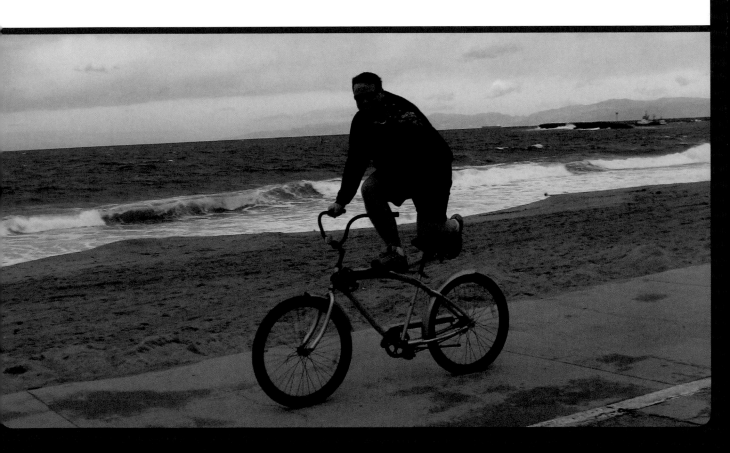

We all know that we need to exercise more to lose weight or to keep it off, so why don't more people do it? As I mentioned, when I decided to audition for a reality show, I was what everyone imagines when you hear "couch potato." I was lying on my couch in front of the TV with a beer (and not my first) in one hand and a near-empty, large bag of chips resting on my (ever-expanding) belly. You want reality TV? Now that's about as real as it gets for a lot of people. It's not my reality anymore, though, and it doesn't have to be yours either. I'm going to tell you what I learned about the importance

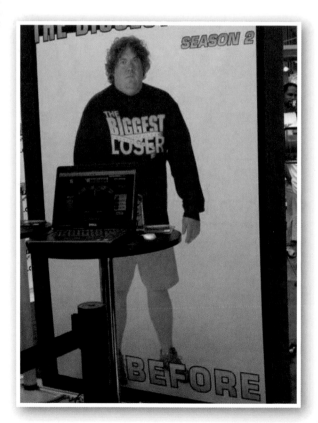 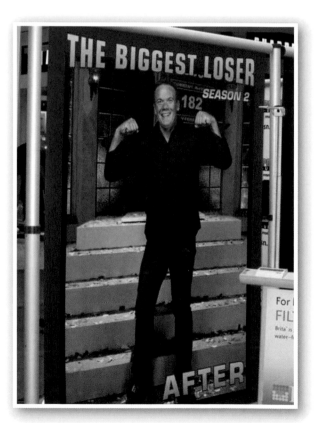

Before and after. Small transformation!

of getting up off the couch and being more physically active (as well as giving up the beer and chips habit).

Keep It Simple, Stupid

The morning after the finale of *The Biggest Loser 2*, I appeared on a slew of national television shows, including *Live with Regis and Kelly* and *The Today Show*. On *The Today Show*, the interviewer asked me the question, "If you could only give one piece of advice on losing weight, what would it be?" My answer was simple, but to the point. I replied, "Close your mouth and move your feet!" How simple could it be? Many people, myself included, think that we have to get a book, read the whole thing, and *then* begin an exercise program. The problem with this way of thinking is that often we never even get around to finishing the book, let alone starting the exercise program that it outlines.

If the book approach doesn't work, often the next step is the "miracle" fat loss pill. You know the pills I'm talking about—the ones that guarantee to help you lose weight fast without you doing a thing, especially not exercising. Let's think about that for a minute. If those pills actually worked, we wouldn't have any obese or overweight people, would we? Beside the fact that many of the "miracle" pills don't work unless you do, most "diet" pills are not regulated by the FDA, so you don't really know what you are putting into your body. While my slogan "Close your mouth and move your feet" doesn't promise to make you thinner without you having to change some of your ways, it does denote the truth: if you implement this slogan, you will get results. The only way to get them, though, is to actually work on improving your lifestyle.

After the show, my father decided to lose a little weight. He was in no way obese; he just wanted to drop a few pounds. I was curious about how he was able to lose weight when he had a full-time job and a life. He didn't even have a big fancy gym. How could any person ever successfully lose weight under those conditions? To find out, I asked my dad his secret. He told me he just pushed away from the table a little sooner, and he went for a walk every day. When his walks got easier, he started to jog, and when the jogging got easier, he began to run. Possibly more amazing than his losing weight is the fact that he has kept it off to this day. Brace yourself for some shocking news: he has maintained the loss by doing the exact same thing that helped him achieve his goal, which was simply closing his mouth and moving his feet.

If eating too much and not moving helped me to gain the weight, why wouldn't the opposite take it back off? I didn't just wake up obese one day; it took a couple years for me to accomplish that feat. For some reason, I truly believed that because I no longer wanted to be fat, I could just wish the weight off. It took going on *The Biggest Loser* for me to implement what I had already known for years was critical to being at a healthy weight, which I was

failing to follow myself. You have to close your mouth and move your feet.

My Workout Secrets from the Biggest Loser Ranch

I'm convinced that my downward spiral started with my perceived failure to achieve my athletic goals. I know I shouldn't have let that be the end of the world, but I really had not learned to create an identity outside of being an athlete. I'd bet a lot of you former athletes know exactly what I'm talking about. At this point in my life, I know how to get into the physical shape of a collegiate athlete or even an Olympian, and you can, too, even if you were never an athlete. Let me tell you what I know about getting fit and then you can do it yourself.

Being on the show certainly gave me access to some excellent personal trainers. They helped me to remember what it was like to work hard. I would have to say that the majority of my time was spent on

"Your body has a set point for your weight that is impossible to bring back down once you gain weight."

Fiction. It's true that your body has a "set point," or a body weight around which you settle and stay most of the time. Many people find that once they lose weight, their bodies try to return to that weight. It's a myth that you can't do anything to permanently lower your set point down to a lower weight after you've gained and then lost weight, though. A lot of your set point has to do with the amount of muscle you have. It's the most active, calorie-requiring tissue in your body, and muscle uses up lots of calories each day, even when you're at rest. One of the few things actually effective for lowering your body's set point is regular physical activity. In fact, most people who lose weight by dieting alone don't actually reset to a lower point, which is why they're even more likely to gain the weight back. Remember that one of the main characteristics of people in the NWCR is that they exercise daily. The older you get, the

➡

more you'll have to fight to maintain or gain muscle mass to keep your metabolism from dropping, and you'll only do so by being as physically active as possible.

endurance workouts, what I call "cardio." It may seem like a no-brainer, but the most important thing, I think, is how hard you do your cardio training, not how long. In gyms and even on the Ranch, I have witnessed people doing hours of cardio and not really getting the results they expect to. A lot of people get frustrated after spending so many hours on the treadmill with so few results. In order to get results fast, I had to get my heart racing.

On the Biggest Loser Ranch, I was able to get in anywhere from four to six hours of cardio training a day, comprised of walking, running, doing the stair climber, jumping rope, swimming, hiking, and more. The key to my success was variety. I tend to easily get bored, but so do a lot of other people I know.

By accepting that it was all right for me to use other workout machines besides just a treadmill, I kept myself from getting burned out.

A fantastic machine to use when you are just starting out is the elliptical strider. This piece of exercise equipment alleviates some of the pressure that can be placed on your knees when you're carrying around extra weight. I think that many people, myself included, tend to jump right into an exercise program without first making a really honest evaluation of themselves and their true exercise capabilities. Let's face it: we all want to get in shape, but most of us don't want to know what terrible shape we're actually in when we start. In order to start the journey toward change, you have to be honest with yourself about where you are when you start.

My first day on the Ranch, my trainer took the whole men's team through a group workout. It was excruciating, and I remember thinking, "What is this woman trying to do? Kill us?" I mean, there I was at 340 pounds, and this lady was working us like we were pro football players. Looking back on that particular moment, I now understand what she was doing. She wasn't trying to hurt us; rather, she was finding out what she had to work with and forcing us to take a realistic look at our actual starting fitness level.

That was a tough day for me. Even though I was obese, I still thought I was in decent shape. I found out that I wasn't. Getting honest with yourself about your physical state, although it may be emotionally painful, is absolutely imperative if true change is going to take place. Although that first day was rough, it did get better for me. Notice that I said "better," not "easier." This is yet another important lesson I learned on the Ranch. When a routine begins to become too easy, it's time to make it more challenging. For example, if you have been working out by walking on the treadmill and you find after a couple of months you're still on the same setting as you were the first day, you probably aren't getting as many benefits from it as you could be by pushing yourself a little harder.

Our bodies have an amazing ability to adapt. It doesn't take long for your body to get used to a routine, and that's the best time to change it up. You may want to know why anyone would want to get to the point of feeling comfortable with a routine, only to make it uncomfortable again. The answer is pretty simple: With an exercise routine that is a little more difficult, you have to push yourself harder, and your fitness level and body weight will both benefit.

On the show, my trainer was a master of reading my body language. She knew when to turn it up a notch and when I really needed to rest. I can't remember how many times I thought I was working hard enough, only to have my trainer crank it up a notch, but trust me when I say that it happened a lot of times. Of course, it became more difficult for me, but I was able to do it. Don't mistake breathing hard for working hard. Although I knew that I was breathing hard, my trainer knew I wasn't working as hard as I could. One of the most important things I have learned from my trainers is that my heart rate is the best way to monitor how hard I am actually working.

So, you could say that there were three really important workout secrets that I took away from my time at the Ranch. The first was that variety truly is the spice of life, and the more activities you add to your exercise routine, the less likely you will be to become bored. Second, change it up. Watch how your body is responding; when an exercise routine becomes too easy, it's time for a change. Add some intensity. Finally, breathing hard is different from working hard! You may just be out of shape. It's better to gauge the intensity of your workout by your heart rate.

The Benefits of Cross-Training and Varying Your Workouts

Another way to become more fit and maximize your weight loss is to do a wide variety of activities. For instance, you may choose to jog or walk briskly for thirty to sixty minutes on Monday, Wednesday, and Friday, but cycle on Tuesdays and swim or row on Saturdays. You should also add in some resistance workouts two to three days a week. The benefits of "cross-training" include keeping your exercise fresh and fun and lowering your risks for developing an overuse ➡

injury that could restrict exercise and impede achieving a higher level of overall fitness. To maximize the calories you burn and weight you lose, try to work out for as long as you can, particularly when you're doing harder workouts. On days that you just feel tired and crappy, give yourself a bit of a break.

You may want to consider varying workout intensities by alternating easier and harder sessions. In fact, recent research indicates that if you do low-volume sprint-interval training, your muscles adapt as well as if you do a whole lot of lower-intensity endurance training. Most competitive athletes vary their training, intermixing some higher-intensity interval training with longer, slower workout days, which allows their bodies to recover better from their intense workouts. You'll also need adequate rest, which includes not just proper amounts of sleep (seven to eight hours a night for most adults), but also enough time between workouts to fully rebuild muscle, restore glycogen, and recuperate. Although easy workouts are a form of "rest" by themselves and do not cause the same level of glycogen depletion or muscle damage as harder sessions, you'll likely benefit from at least one day of true rest a week, a day on which you only do your normal daily activities.

A Typical Day at the Ranch—Sort of

One of the questions I hear on a regular basis is, "What was a typical day on the Ranch like?" I really do have to work hard to contain myself because *there was nothing typical about being on the Ranch!* I don't think people can understand how atypical it was. The results, the work, and the lifestyle on the Ranch can only be understood by the folks who were there. That being said, I'll do my best to describe what it was like to be in such an abnormal environment.

My "typical" day on the Ranch began with a morning cardio session. I was usually sore in the morning, so a brisk walk was my way to get ready for the day, ease some of my soreness, and get my body moving. Some people on the show liked to get going early in the morning, but I am not a morning person and didn't begin my first workout until around 10:00 AM. I think it is important for everyone to work out at the time(s) that work best for you. If you hate to get up in the morning and know that you won't get up at 5:00 AM to work out, then don't set yourself up to fail. You'll just end up discouraged and disappointed in yourself. Instead, set a time that you can stick to.

After my morning workout (usually a walk), I came back and had lunch, a hamburger mix that I prepared using onions, garlic, and cilantro. I added a little mayo and some mustard after it was cooked. It was nothing fancy, but it gave me the energy that I needed for the rest of the day. I ate almost the same thing every day I was there. On days that I was tired of that menu, I typically prepared some low-fat chicken patties on the grill.

After lunch, I relaxed a little bit before my workout with my trainer. I saved my energy for that workout because to me, it was my most important workout of the day. Most of the time, I began with a run on the treadmill, usually at level five for five to fifteen minutes. It worked well to warm up my body and to prepare me mentally for the next hour or so with my trainer.

After that, I did a strength workout, usually a circuit session, since I was trying not to increase muscle (because of its weight). I wanted to maintain the muscle I already had and benefit from cardio training (and calorie usage) at the same time. (For those of you who have no idea what a "circuit" is, it's when you lift weights by moving quickly from one resistance exercise to the next in order to keep your heart rate up.) As recommended by my trainer, I did my circuits using lighter weights and a higher number of repetitions. In between lifting exercises, I often did an exercise like light jogging in place to keep my heart rate up while my trainer got the next station ready.

A typical circuit went something like this. From the treadmill I went to the chest press, and after about fifteen reps I did "mountain climbers" for about thirty to sixty seconds before doing fifteen to twenty tricep dips. The dips were followed by squat jumps for another thirty seconds to one minute. The next station was chest flys (anywhere from ten to fifteen reps) on a stability ball. Next, I lay on my stomach and rose up to the plank position, which I held for thiry to sixty seconds. Then I did tricep press downs (fifteen reps), followed by up to a minute of high knees, which involves alternately bringing my knees up toward my chest as fast as possible—kind of like running in place, but a lot harder to do. After completing all of that, I started all over again.

I didn't do a lot of lifting with my legs on the Ranch. If you look at the workout I did closely, you can I was focusing on two areas, my torso and my arms. In the periods between the resistance exercises, I worked on other muscle groups, specifically my legs and abs, but not using weights. I alternated groups from day to day, usually doing two circuit days and then having a "rest day" of just cardio, followed by two more circuit days. If I did chest and triceps on one day, I targeted my back and biceps the next. Keep in mind that I only did this workout after I had built up the capacity to do it safely. If you're just starting, I would recommend stopping to rest between sets. After my weight session, I always tried to get some protein into my body, usually in the form of a shake with only 110 calories and many nutrients. After my snack, which was soon after my workout session, I simply took time to rest.

The next session later on was another cardio workout. I love the stair machine; nearly every day I did it for thirty to forty five minutes at a difficult level to keep my heart rate high. Afterward, I ate some supper (that's dinner for those of you not familiar with the lingo of the Midwest), usually consisting of a steak with a salad or some vegetables—again nothing fancy, but it was what my body worked well with. After finishing, I rested for a while and then got another cardio session in. Many times I did a swimming workout or jumped rope. After that last workout, I literally fell into

bed, fully exhausted after a typical day at the Ranch.

It wasn't a very exciting existence. I varied my cardio exercises, but for the most part my schedule was very consistent. Sundays I considered my rest day. On that day, I went on a long hike in the mountains, usually for at least four hours. It was a good change of pace and broke the monotony of working out in the gym. It was also a good way to clear my head and get myself prepared for the upcoming week.

One of the things I forgot to mention—and probably the most important detail of my "typical" Ranch day—is the fact that I *always* had my big cup or a bottle of water with me. My favorite cup was filled with ice water. Truly, drinking water is the thing that helped me the most with my weight loss. If I was getting hungry and felt a binge coming on, I simply drank a glass of water and, surprisingly, I always felt satisfied.

I was on the Ranch for three months, and nearly every day was the same. My life strangely resembled the Bill Murray movie *Groundhog Day*. Do you remember that movie? In it, Bill Murray's character woke up and repeated the previous day over and over. It got to the point that he knew exactly what was going to happen every second of every day. The Ranch was my own version of that movie. Movies all have an ending, and mine eventually did, too. When my time on the Ranch was over, I had to go home, where things were definitely *not* like *Groundhog Day*.

Post-Ranch, but Still Losing

After I got home from the Ranch, it took quite some time before I even felt comfortable leaving my house; I had six more months to lose weight on my own before the final weigh-in. On the Ranch, I had been living in a bubble where all I had to do was work out, watch my diet, and focus on losing weight. Now I was back in the real world with no trainer, no rules, real temptations, and equally real responsibilities. Not

only that, but I was back to where many of my troubles had begun. I was scared, probably as scared as I had been in my entire life. All of the safety and security I felt at the Ranch stayed behind in California, which didn't do me much good halfway across the country in Iowa. I needed a game plan—in a hurry. A friend of mine owned a construction company and let me work part-time for him so that I could keep up with my workouts. My schedule wasn't quite as intense as it was on the Ranch, but it still wasn't all that typical.

My day started off with breakfast, which was usually one cup of cereal mixed with a container of yogurt. After breakfast, I headed off to work. If I was able to, I rode my bike the seventeen miles to the job site with my work clothes in a backpack. I was eager to be the gopher at work, carrying lumber, shingles, or plywood wherever needed. I was glad to do it because it kept me moving all day long. I always brought my lunch with me, and it was pretty much the same: a salad

"Exercising always makes you lose weight faster."

Fiction. About the only thing that exercise can't always do is decrease your body weight faster than dieting alone. When you cut back on your calorie intake, what you lose is a combination of body fat, muscle mass, and water weight. By exercising, you actually keep and even gain some muscle mass, which is good for revving up your metabolism and making your body use more calories on a daily basis. The downside of retaining or gaining muscle—if it really can be considered a negative—is that muscle is denser than body fat and, thus, it weighs more. As a result, with exercise you can lose fat while retaining or gaining muscle; even though you're losing body fat, your weight on the scales may change very little (or even rise slightly at first). Over time, though, you're sure to see some body weight losses, even when you're gaining muscle, so just keep with it and stay motivated by concentrating more on your measurements and how your clothes fit than your weight.

with a cut-up grilled chicken breast or some type of deli meat. After work, I got a cardio workout in, either a bike ride home or a run outside. Supper was usually a steak or some chicken on the grill with some vegetables. Afterward, I relaxed a while before my last workout of the day, which was a one-hour stationary bike ride. Then I retired for the night.

I was not a big fan of the gym, and I spent much of my time outside simply being active. On the weekends during the summer, I went water skiing or mountain biking. When fall came, wrestling practice started. I had been an assistant coach at Cornell College in Mount Vernon (Iowa) the previous year, and head coach Mike Duroe allowed me to come back and work out with the team, joining their workouts as if I were one of the student athletes. I feel that my wrestling workouts were what gave me the advantage over my competitors on the show; they really kept me focused on my goal and mentally tough as well as physically. You sure don't want a bunch of college athletes a lot younger than you thinking you're a loser, so you try harder and stay tougher.

I also went back to Carver Hawkeye Arena at the University of Iowa to relive my college wrestling drill—running up and down the notorious stairs of Carver. I can't put into words what it's like to run those stairs, but it is a widely held belief that the

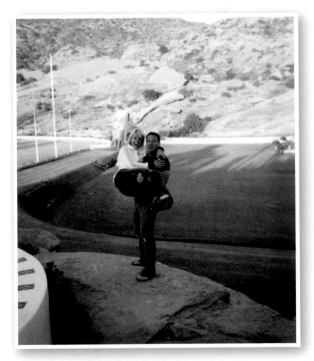

Suzy and I on the Biggest Loser Ranch.

stairs are a big reason for the Iowa wrestlers' great conditioning and success. They are brutal! As I ran them, I couldn't help but think of how different my wrestling career would have been at Iowa had I trained that hard when I had actually had the chance. Those thoughts helped to motivate me to work even harder. I didn't want to be left with "what ifs" after this opportunity on *The Biggest Loser*.

That's how it went for the nine months of my life that I was on the show. I didn't go out much, I wasn't very social, and my life was completely consumed by dieting and exercising. Looking back, though, it was all worth it.

How to Start Moving Your Feet More

At one point during my weight loss journey, I found myself complaining to my brother about how long the weight loss process was taking. My brother, who had lost over one hundred pounds himself, said something that has stuck with me to this day. I have shared this with thousands of people during my talks. It is quite simple, but often overlooked when we start a weight loss program. My brother said, "You didn't put all that weight on overnight. Why do you expect it to come off overnight, idiot?" First, let me say my brother and I have different endearing terms for each other. Second, duh, it makes sense, doesn't it? In all my travels, I have yet to meet someone who says, "You know, Matt, it's the darndest thing. I went to bed last night and I weighed 185. Now, you're not going to believe this, but this morning when I got on the scale, I weighed 350! Just like that, overnight, I put on 165 pounds!"

If someone walked up to you and made that statement, you would look at him like he was crazy, yet many of us actually tell ourselves that story every day. It starts out with, "Man, I need to lose a couple pounds," and then becomes, "Man, I need to lose about ten pounds." This statement progresses to

"It's possible to burn a significant number of calories by just standing more and fidgeting."

Fact. Standing, talking, and fidgeting use up extra calories and can make a difference in your body weight. In tracking lean and obese people for ten days, researchers observed that the overweight, self-proclaimed couch potatoes stayed seated for about two and a half hours longer per day than their leaner counterparts, spending about 350 fewer calories per day—the caloric equivalent of about thirty-six pounds a year. Just staying on your feet more can have a beneficial impact on your body weight, so stand up while you're reading this book!

As for fidgeting, that falls under the category known as NEAT, or non-exercise activity thermogenesis (heat production, a byproduct of metabolism), which is the cumulative amount of energy you expend through all the activities of daily living. While it is highly variable among individuals (some of us may be genetically wired to fidget), there is mounting evidence to suggest that NEAT is critical in determining your susceptibility to gaining excess body weight. So feel free to fidget while you're reading as well.

Dr. Sheri's Tips for Moving More Every Day

- Add as many additional steps as possible (a minimum of 2,000) every day by walking whenever and wherever you can.
- Whenever you have ten free minutes, walk around instead of sitting down—or at least stay up on your feet.
- Always take the stairs instead of the elevator or escalator; if going up is too hard at first, start with going down.
- Do more physical chores around the house, such as cleaning, sweeping, mopping, vacuuming, and washing dishes (even if you have a dishwasher).
- Mow your lawn with a push mower, rake leaves in your yard, shovel snow, or do some gardening.
- Go shopping for groceries or window-shopping at the nearest mall.
- Put on some music and dance around your house.
- Set up a basketball hoop in your driveway, or walk to the nearest neighborhood school and use theirs.
- Take the dog out for a daily walk (it needs exercise, too!).
- Get up and move around for a few minutes after every thirty minutes of a sedentary activity to increase your daily activity levels.

- Walk around or simply stand up while talking on the telephone instead of sitting down.
- Hide the remotes for the TV, stereo, and other devices so that you have to get up occasionally to change them by hand.
- Walk in place, dance, move around, or even just stand up while watching TV, starting with the commercial breaks and working up to longer periods of time.
- Limit your TV and computer use to no more than two hours per day, or at least reduce your use by a minimum of thirty minutes daily.

the point where we finally say, "Man, what has happened to me? When did I gain all this weight?" By then, rather than trying to work off the weight, we begin to try and wish it off. The point of the preceding rant is this: if it took more than a day, a week, or a year to get to the point of needing to lose a large amount of weight, then chances are more than likely that it will take a similar amount of time to lose it again.

I had such a rare opportunity to be in the situation that I was in while losing my weight. I did it on reality TV, but what is someone supposed to do in real life? How are people supposed to find time to lose a large amount of weight? When I gained my weight, I did it by having a little extra food here, a couple extra drinks there, until it became a habit to eat and drink too much. What if you turn it around the other direction? For instance, when it came to increasing my exercise, I found a walk here, some weights there worked for me, and eventually exercising became a habit. So, how do we find the time to lose weight? We do it by making a few small changes at a time and losing a little at a time.

If you are capable, the first step is moving more, which is exactly that: moving more. I am seriously just talking about walking around the house or getting up to change the channel instead of using the remote. Try a push mower instead of a riding one. How about this? Go outside and play with your kids. If you don't have kids, go outside and play like a kid. When you feel comfortable, head out for a walk. Be realistic, though: if the most exercise you

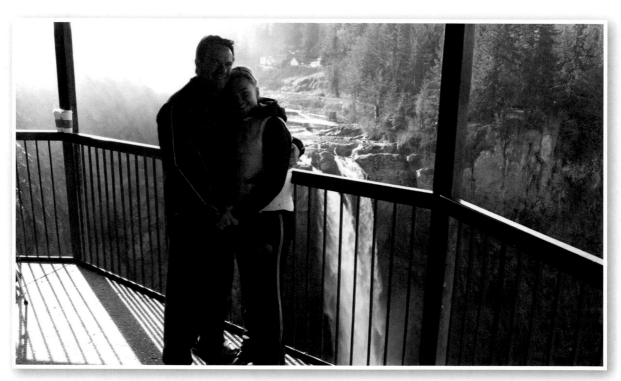

Hiking at Snoqualmie Falls in Washington—one of our favorite places.

have had in the last several years is getting up to pay the pizza delivery person, don't sign up for the Chicago Marathon just yet. Your first walk may be just down to the end of the block. When that starts to get easy, add another block and then another, and before long you will be seeing your neighborhood and eventually your whole town from the sidewalk.

One of the things I hear at almost every speaking event I do is the following: "I'm too embarrassed to go for a walk. I'm afraid people will make fun of me." I have to agree that is a very valid statement—but only if you are not serious about starting an exercise program. To those people I say, "Chances are people are already making fun of you. At least now you are doing something about it."

The real question to ask yourself is why you would let someone whom you have never met and who obviously doesn't care about you affect your life and your opportunity to improve it? If you are afraid of being ridiculed for your weight, then imagine what will happen if you stick to a healthy diet plan and go for a walk every day, adding distance as you are able to for a year. Visualize what you will look like in a year or two. Do you still see someone who is being made fun of? I seriously doubt it. Most of us focus on the negative aspects of beginning an exercise program rather than visualizing the successes that we are going to make happen in our lives farther down the road.

Losing weight really is relatively simple. There are thousands of books out there that use difficult formulas to calculate what you should eat, or when you should eat. Let me sum them all up for you so that you never have to buy another one: eat fewer calories than you are now and move more. In essence, close your mouth and move your feet. I don't know why it took me so long to figure it out.

Walking Counts as Aerobic Exercise?

When it comes to weight loss, walking may be one of the most overlooked forms of exercise. It's hard to imagine the benefits of such a seemingly simple exercise; every time you see a show like *The Biggest Loser*, you see people running to exhaustion or doing kickboxing with sweat just rolling down their faces. While in no way am I saying you shouldn't strive to achieve that level of fitness, when you're starting out, an old-fashioned walk is a good place to begin.

When we were kids, many of us used to walk to school. Although at the time it didn't seem like much, it was a great way to

Fact or Fiction?

"It's healthier to be fat and fit than thin and unfit."

Fact. While it's best to be both leaner and fit, it is entirely possible to be fit even if you're still overweight, and your health will benefit more from fitness than weight loss. When you exercise regularly, you lower your risk for many health problems, including heart disease, obesity, hypertension, type 2 diabetes, certain cancers, and other metabolic disorders. Much of what we attribute to getting older—muscle atrophy or loss of flexibility in joints—really results from disuse and inactivity over time. Thus, regular exercise can keep you looking and feeling younger for longer and even greatly reduce your risk of having health problems.

How Much Exercise Does It Take to Get Fit?

How much and what types of exercises do you need to do to reach an acceptable minimal level of fitness? According to updated physical activity guidelines released jointly in 2007 by the American College of Sports Medicine (ACSM) and the American Heart Association (AHA), all healthy adults ages eighteen to sixty-five years need to engage in moderate-intensity aerobic physical activity for at least thirty minutes five days each week or vigorous aerobic physical activity for at least twenty minutes on three days. In addition, adults will benefit from performing activities that maintain or increase muscular strength and endurance (i.e., resistance training) for at least two days each week. You should plan to do such activities in addition to your usual light-intensity activities of daily living, such as casual walking, grocery shopping, or any physical activities that last less than ten minutes, like walking to the parking lot or taking out the trash. If you're over sixty-five, do all of the above, add extra focus on maintaining your flexibility, and do extra balance training to prevent falling.

start off the school day. You had probably just had a reasonable breakfast, headed out the door to meet your friend who also walked to school, and talked about the day ahead. When you got to class, you were ready and eager to learn. That's not the end of it, though. After school, you met up with your friend and headed home, again on foot. Along the way you probably talked about your day, which girls you liked and which ones you didn't, upcoming projects, plans for the weekend—the topics and the conversation were limitless.

I don't know about you, but for me this scenario continued through my junior high school years, and then *it* happened. I moved up to high school and suddenly walking to school wasn't cool anymore. In fact, walking *anywhere* was about as uncool as you could get. I truly believe that as far as big moments in our young lives went, being in high school was one of the biggest reasons many of us started to think walking

was no longer beneficial. I remember the day I got my driver's license. Not only was I convinced that I would never have to walk anywhere again, but I tried my hardest to make it happen.

I am married again, and my wife and I have our first child. A big part of our lives is that we try to go—now brace yourself—for a *walk* every day. Walking together not only allows us to get in an extra cardio session, but it also gives us a chance to communicate with each other. Just like in elementary school, we are walking buddies who use the time to share how our day went or make plans. What a great opportunity! In a world where people in relationships are always lamenting their lack of communication and how they wish they could spend more time together, imagine what would happen if people simply took a walk together each and every day. The number of obese people would likely dwindle, and perhaps the number of failed relationships and marriages would decline as well.

Alternate Exercises to Stay Off Your Feet

If you have arthritic knees or hips, which are more common when you're overweight or older, walking may be too uncomfortable or painful. Your best option is to try non-weight-bearing activities, such as "walking" in a pool (with or without a flotation belt around your waist), aqua aerobics, lap swimming, recumbent stationary cycling, upper-body exercises, seated aerobic workouts, and resistance activities.

A wide selection of videotapes and DVDs demonstrating various physical activities, including exercise routines to be done in a chair or wheelchair, are available from a variety of sources. You can find aerobic workouts, strength training, flexibility moves, yoga, and more. In addition to locating them at local sporting-goods stores and national chains, check online sources for workout videos and DVDs that you can do, even seated ones like Jodi Stolove's *Chair Dancing through the Decades* and *Chair Dancing around the World*.

My Typical Weekly Workout Nowadays

I'll be the first one to admit that my daily workout schedule is not that exciting, but it works for me. I function better with a set routine; that way I'm more likely to follow through with it on a daily basis. Although I did a lot more exercise when I was trying to win the show, I'm more moderate nowadays because I have other things in my life that are equally important, including my wife and son and career. I'll give you an idea of how much exercise I do on a daily basis now, though.

On Mondays, I go for a forty-five-minute walk at a good pace in the morning, lift weights at 3:00 PM, and then wrestle for up to an hour or so at 4:30. Sometimes, I substitute a thirty- to sixty-minute cardio workout for wrestling, using one of the fitness machines in the gym. On Tuesdays, I do the same routine. Wednesdays I just go for a walk and wrestle, without lifting. On Thursdays and Fridays, I follow the same workout schedule as I do the first two days of the week.

Here's a list of the resistance training exercises that I usually do on my lifting days:

- Legs: Lunges, sumo squats, jump squats, step-ups, calf raises, leg press, leg extensions, leg curls, leg curls on stability ball
- Chest: Chest press, incline press, dumbbell flys, wide push-ups, cable crossovers
- Back: Lat pull-downs, seated rows, pull-ups, modified pull-ups
- Shoulders: Lateral raises, shoulder press, low pull
- Biceps: Curls (several variations)
- Triceps: Tricep press-downs (variations), skull crushers, dips, and modified dips

Weekends are a little different for me, exercise-wise. Saturdays, I usually go hiking on a mountain trail for about three hours. I love getting out and spending time with nature, and hiking is a great way to do that. If I can't hit the trails for some reason, I substitute a hilly walk that day. On Sundays, I spend more time with my family, going for a long walk with Suzy and Rex. It's like my rest day, but I'm still being physically active—it's just more relaxed than my workouts on other days.

Resistance Training "Dos" and "Don'ts"

Do:

- Use resistance training to exercise all parts of your body (upper and lower body, abs, and lower back) two to three nonconsecutive days per week.
- Start each workout session with exercises that use multiple muscle groups first (e.g., thighs), and then isolate smaller muscle groups (such as the hamstrings in the back of your thighs) with other exercises.
- Equally train opposing muscle groups around joints, such as biceps and triceps in your upper arm, to avoid injuries.
- Complete at least one set per exercise with eight to twelve repetitions to complete exhaustion (or more reps for circuit or lighter training). ➡

- Exhale fully as you work against or lift the resistance and inhale during the return to the starting position.
- Rest for two to three minutes between each set of the same exercise (when doing two or more).
- Use your full range of motion around each joint during exercises.
- Allow yourself at least forty-eight hours between workouts on specific parts of your body (i.e., upper body, lower body, etc.) to recuperate.
- Stretch during and/or after resistance training workouts to achieve greater strength gains.
- Initially focus on good body mechanics and technique, and then add more weight or resistance—slowly, to avoid injury.
- Find a workout center with resistance training machines or free weights to push yourself with once your strength increases.

Don't:

- Fully lock your knees when your legs are supporting the weight (or your elbows during upper-body work).
- Pick up any weights from the floor by bending over with straight legs (to avoid low back strain).

- Fatigue your abs before completing other exercises, particularly when using free weights or resistance bands.
- Work out with exercises that focus on the same muscle groups two consecutive days.
- Ever hold your breath while doing resistance work.
- Do sit-ups with your back straight (rather than curling forward).
- Sacrifice your form just to add more weight, resistance, or reps.
- Continue with an exercise if you feel a sharp or immediate pain in any joint or muscle; it could be indicative of an acute injury.

"Use it or lose it."

Fact. Strength training is absolutely critical if you want to maintain the amount of muscle you currently have, gain more, or prevent loss of muscle and strength as you age. Being sedentary also accelerates your loss of muscle mass, so it truly is a case of "Use it or lose it." Although aerobic training can help, only the muscle fibers that you recruit and use regularly will be maintained over time. Unfortunately, moderate walking does not bring all of your muscle fibers into play, only the slower and intermediate ones in most cases. Only more intense workouts or intervals can recruit the rest, so you should plan on doing some resistance and/or sprint training to preserve your faster (stronger) muscle fibers. Resistance training can increase muscle mass, which revs up your metabolism and helps you control your body weight better, not to mention enhancing your self-esteem and body satisfaction. Once you start training, your strength can increase significantly in as short a time as one to two weeks (from neural changes, which occur before increases in muscle size), which is motivating. Furthermore, major strength gains and muscle fiber retention occur even if you just train one day a week, so get on it!

Do It for Your Heart

Even if you don't end up as fit as an Olympian, to save your heart and improve your health you should consider increasing your fitness level. If you watched the show, you may remember that during that time I lost my uncle to heart disease at a young age. His passing, though, could have been prevented if he had lived a healthier lifestyle. What's worse, at my heaviest weight, I started showing early signs of heart problems—before I even reached the big 3-0! In chapter 7, I'll tell you a lot more about the health problems I was having before I changed my lifestyle and started exercising and eating better foods. Suffice it to say, if I hadn't turned my life around when I did, I probably wouldn't still be alive to tell my story to you or anyone else.

"It's always good to drink lots of water when you're working out."

Fiction. It's actually easier to harm yourself with excessive fluid intake than with dehydration during exercise. If you drink too much water and other fluids during exercise, you'll increase your risk of diluting the sodium levels in your bloodstream, potentially causing a medical condition known as hyponatremia, or water intoxication, which raises your risk for seizures, coma, and even death. To avoid over-hydrating, only begin drinking when you actually feel thirsty. Drinking before meals, however, is recommended, because the extra fluid in your stomach will make you feel fuller and keep you from eating as much at that meal. Starting your meal with a broth-based soup is also good for the same reason.

Dr. Sheri's Tips for Preventing and Treating Injuries Caused by Exercising Too Hard

No matter what physical activity you choose, start out slowly and progress gradually, using pain as your guide. If you ever feel acute pain while working out, stop the activity immediately. If the pain persists, treat it with the standard RICE approach (rest, ice, compression, elevation), so well known to athletes and their trainers. Taking over-the-counter pain medications like aspirin, ibuprofen, or Aleve can also help. If it doesn't get better within a few days, consider consulting with a doctor to make sure the injury does not require other treatments.

To prevent chronic, or overuse, injuries, focus on strategies like alternating your workout intensities (mild, moderate, and heavy) and taking enough rest time to recuperate between workouts. Varying your exercises also helps prevent such injuries, which are often the result of overstressing your body with repeated heavy workouts, especially if you're doing the same activity over and over again. You can often tell that you have "overuse syndrome" if you start having frequent and lasting colds, chronic tiredness, and numerous or recurring joint and muscle injuries, including stress fractures in bones and tendonitis, or inflamed tendons (e.g., rotator cuff tendonitis in your shoulder that makes it painful to lift your arm straight out to the side). At least one day of rest a week is vitally important, even if on that day you do a different activity or just some low-intensity walking. Another key to preventing injuries is doing varied types of activities, the cross-training idea mentioned previously.

As for muscle soreness, it's caused by overloading your muscles, particularly during the "eccentric" phase (also known as doing "negatives") of muscle contraction, when the muscle is lengthening. Examples of some activities that can cause delayed-onset muscle soreness (DOMS) that typically peaks forty-eight to seventy-two hours after the damaging workout are downhill running (your quads will get sore), heavy resistance training, and new or unusual activities. Doing some mild activity like walking when your legs are sore, stretching, having a gentle massage, getting into a hot tub, and taking anti-inflammatory medications like aspirin and ibuprofen can help alleviate the pain and discomfort you are feeling, but the best healer is simply time. Your body responds with "stress" proteins that it builds into the repaired muscles, which at least partially protect you against becoming that sore again for the next six to eight weeks.

CHAPTER 5

A Dating, Sex, and Love Guide for the Overweight

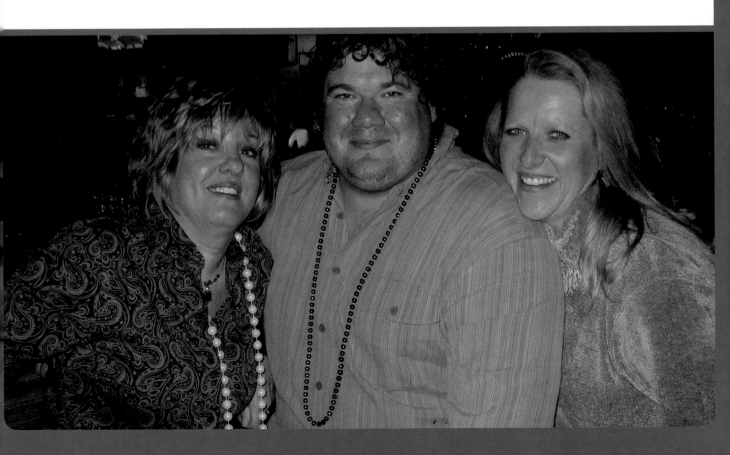

Whether you blame it on an instinct linked to the survival of the species or something else, there is just no getting around the fact that most of us are driven to couple with someone, usually someone of the opposite sex. The dating game is a hard one for us guys to figure out (when am I really supposed to buy her flowers, and why did she burst into tears when I gave her chocolate?), but being overweight changes all of the unwritten rules in ways that I don't think I fully realized until I lost some weight.

Dating as an Obese Man

Dating is hard enough when you are a good-looking, fit guy. I know firsthand how hard it is when you are obese. I dated a lot when I was younger and fit. I couldn't figure out why it was so hard when I was big. After all, I had a "great personality," or so said the girls that I was interested in who had no interest in me. Stop me if you have ever heard this one: "You are like a brother to me." What a load of crap.

Let me share a personal story with you. I decided I would try the Internet dating world, so I signed up, got my profile, and began to search the Web for my true love. I was truthful. I talked about all the things I loved to do and said I was a former college athlete, even mentioning that I was a big guy with broad shoulders and a "little extra" weight (I was only three hundred pounds then). That was how I saw myself at the time.

One night I got home and saw that I had a message from a potential date. Of course, I looked at her picture first and then her profile. After all I didn't want to date some big, fat girl. She looked pretty good, and I contacted her right away. After a few notes back and forth, we found out that we had a lot of common interests and decided to meet in person. I got to her place and sat outside for a minute, thinking to myself, "I can't believe you are about to do this. What if she is some big, fat girl or a freak?" I walked up to the door, sucked in my gut, and knocked. Imagine her surprise when the guy with "a little extra weight" she was about to go out with that night turned out to be a five-foot-ten-inch, three hundred-pounder. The look on her face said it all.

Everything that I had been thinking about her, she had been thinking about me, only she was the one whose fears had been justified. I knew she was uncomfortable, so I told her she didn't have to go out to dinner if she didn't want to. She was nice enough to agree to still go out, but it turned out to be a very uncomfortable date for both of us. I took her to a very nice restaurant, and we made it through some forced conversation and a little bit of dinner before she excused herself to go to the bathroom. When she got back, she said she wasn't feeling very well. I suggested we call it a night, and I took her home and dropped her off. To this day, I'm pretty sure it wasn't the food that made her ill and that it was probably just me. Needless to say, that was my first and last Internet dating experience.

Looking back on that night, I find it quite comical, but at the time I was devastated. I think it was at that point that I finally realized I did indeed have a weight problem and that appearance truly is the most important thing to some people. I am a nice guy, and I actually do have a great personality, as well as a big heart. Unfortunately, those qualities don't appear to be important in the dating world. When it comes down to it, people do and will continue to base compatibility on looks. Being obese or overweight doesn't help in that area.

How to Make a Good First Impression Despite Your Weight

Don't judge others based on their appearance. It's what's on the inside that's important. Beauty is only skin deep. Yeah, right! Whether we choose to believe it or not, we are all judged daily based solely on our physical appearance. Maybe the only cliché that

"Women are more willing to date overweight men than the reverse."

Fact. When it comes to dating an overweight person, men and women are not equally discriminatory. In one study, researchers found that although young women are more concerned about their weight than men are about theirs, women are more willing than men to date an overweight person of the opposite sex. In other words, dating someone of the "right" weight is much more important to young men than women, and the women are more concerned about being at that ideal weight themselves. However, younger women are more likely to consider themselves overweight and have more stringent body weight ideals than men have about women. Similarly, among college-aged men and women, men who are told by their partners to gain weight and women who are advised to lose weight report less satisfaction in their relationships.

we hear regularly that holds any amount of water is the good ol' "You never get a second chance to make a first good impression." The fact of the matter, regardless of what you choose to believe on this topic, is that first impressions are usually based on another person's idea of beauty or attractiveness.

Even when I was 350 pounds, I still formed opinions of people I didn't know at all on a personal level, based solely on how they looked. If I saw a person bigger than me, I thought, "Man, he must be really lazy," or "How did she let herself get like that?" Even today I still find myself thinking about how much better-looking a person would be if he or she lost a little, or a lot, of weight.

If everyone thinks like that, how can a person who doesn't look like a fitness model ever make a first good impression? One of the things that I speak about at my seminars is the importance of knowing yourself all the way to the core. That level of self-knowledge gives you confidence, a strong characteristic that shines through. Even the most timid of

people will come out of their shells when doing something that they feel confident about. So the first step in making a good impression is to be confident. Be confident in yourself, the talents you have, the knowledge you possess, and the things you have to offer that no one else on this earth can.

Confidence is the offspring of preparation. Confident people become that way by doing what's necessary to be ready to handle any situation that they face. When I used to wrestle, I was always confident because I was well-prepared. I knew that I was well-conditioned because I had done my running, that I was technically ready because I had spent hours working on my moves, and that I was mentally on top of my game because I was always spending time visualizing my success.

Another key is to be physical. I'm not talking about walking into a room, walking up to someone, and pushing him in the chest. No, I'm talking about being physically active. I have found that in my own life, by simply being active I carry myself differently. Even if you aren't in great shape, knowing that you are doing something to improve it can make you feel better about yourself. When I am working out, I can see differences in my face (it looks thinner) in only a couple of workouts. As your body image improves, your attitude will, too, and that will spill over into other aspects of your life.

Another trick is to take more care in your appearance. Tuck in your shirt! When I weighed 350, leaving it untucked did *not* make me look thinner, despite what I wanted to believe. It just made me look even bigger and more like a slob who didn't take pride in his own appearance. The simple act of tucking in your shirt shows that you care what you look like. Along the same lines, pull up your pants. I know from experience that it is hard to find pants that fit well when you have a fifty-inch waist and a thirty-two-inch inseam. However, it doesn't cost that much to have your pants hemmed, which should take care of the frumpy look.

Another thing that can help your pants fit better is simply wearing a belt.

Next, stand up straight! Hunched shoulders and a hanging head only make you look bigger. When a person walks in a room with his head held high, shoulders back, and chest out, he exudes confidence and makes it known that he cares about himself and that he has something positive to offer.

Finally, take a shower, and do it often. I sweat a lot now, but I sweated even more when I was obese. To make a good first impression, you have to be clean and well-groomed. A shower, a clean shave, deodorant, and a little cologne can make you feel confident in your looks (and your body odor).

Love and Marriage as a Pre-Obese and Obese Man

I got married for the first time in 2001. I was briefly married to a girl that I met at the University of Iowa. She was a cross-country runner, I was a wrestler, and we both thought

"You influence who you are by what you think about yourself."

Fact. Your own perceptions of who you think you are largely determine what you do and how you feel about yourself. If you have a negative self-image, you're likely to fail at whatever you try to do, while having a positive self-image plays a large role in whether you succeed in life. Being positive is an armor against negative messages and a powerful force to help you gain self-confidence in everything you do. If your self-esteem is strong, even some weight gain or regain is not likely to completely destroy your ability to continue to believe in your self-worth.

Where do your positive and negative messages come from? The comments and criticisms that you receive as you're growing up from parents, relatives, teachers, and friends can all have a powerful influence on your self-image. Particularly when heard often enough, these messages are replayed in our minds unless or until we consciously take action to change them. Sometimes just recognizing your self-messages can be the first step in changing or improving

➡

them. At some point, you have to realize that you and you alone have the power to decide whether to make the same mistakes over and simply follow the same life path and lifestyle with which you're most familiar. You have choices, and although changing those messages is hard work, you can do it—and improve your self-image in the process.

Learning How to Accept Compliments (Especially If You're Not Used to Them)

- Give yourself positive messages and real compliments.
- Praise yourself for what you do right, and do this as often as you can—repetition helps counter your instinctive reaction to reject them.
- Make a list of the things you like about yourself, and come up with a list of positive adjectives to describe yourself (like funny, happy, loving, etc.).

- If making a positive list about yourself is too hard, come up with one about someone else you know and see if any of it applies to you as well (and be honest with yourself).

- Try to find the compassion and love within you to offer yourself these healing messages.

- Allow yourself to feel compassion and love for the hurt child that exists inside of you.

- Relieve yourself of any guilt or blame that you were led to feel by your parents, especially if they let you know that they were disappointed in you for any reason.

- Ask someone you care about and trust to tell you many things that he or she likes about and values in you.

- Practice seeing the positives in yourself to learn to accept compliments; you have to find and accept them yourself before you can accept approval from another person.

- Find multiple ways to give yourself positive messages about yourself, and do so as often as you can.

- Write down the positive things other people have said about you in the past, and read these over from time to time. ➡

- Pay attention to how you feel when someone gives you a compliment; if your automatic response is to reject it as not being true or applying to you, stop yourself from saying so.
- Tell yourself that you deserve to feel good about yourself.

about how lucky our future kids would be to get "athletic" genes from both of us. The first years of our courtship were pretty good. We got along well and were very active together. But as the relationship progressed, I found myself becoming more and more sedentary. I think she handled it pretty well for a while, but eventually my laziness wore on her nerves. I don't ever remember her coming right out and telling me I needed to lose weight, but the signs were there.

As her attraction for me diminished, my insecurities increased. I began to drink more and spend less time around her. Soon, I found myself drinking a whole lot and eating even more. On some gut level, I think I knew we shouldn't get married,

and I think she did, too. I have to say that aside from the fact that I was certain no one else would love me the way I had become (which was one reason I went ahead and married her), I was afraid to call off the wedding because all of the preparations had been made. I thought about how embarrassing it would be to have to tell everyone we had decided not to get married. I guess getting divorced within a year of being married seemed less embarrassing to me somehow.

The fatter I got, the more I took it out on my wife at that time. She was a thin, attractive woman, and I would find myself getting upset that she stayed so thin while my weight was steadily progressing upward. To make myself feel better, I would pick fights with her to try and validate my own insecurities (at least, I see now that's what I was doing). When she said mean things back, I had succeeded in proving to myself that *she* was the reason I was miserable. We tried a few times to make things work. I would start working out again, and we would have conversations about how we missed the way we use to be, only to get back together and find out that neither of us had really changed, nor did we want to.

Looking back on that season of my life, I realize a couple of things. First, you can't love someone else if you can't love and respect yourself first. For years after our divorce, I blamed my ex-wife for the failure of our marriage. I could only think of all the things that she had done to hurt me and make me miserable. I felt that because of her I could never love again and would never be loved by another woman. It wasn't until years later that I understood that I had hurt her equally as much and that the failure of our marriage was not all her fault. I was as much to blame because of my lack of respect for and care of myself; our failure wasn't all due to what I perceived as her lack of caring for me during my depression. In essence, I expected to get all of my love from someone else rather than from myself. It is unfair to put that much of a burden on anyone; it is truly unreasonable to expect one human being to fulfill another.

After being on *The Biggest Loser 2*, I realized that as bad as things had seemed when I was married, it was definitely in both of our best interests to no longer be together. At that time of my life, I was not capable of giving any part of myself to anyone, so to try and force a relationship to work only would have made both of our lives even unhappier. One day after the show was over, I called my ex-wife and apologized for the way I had been when we were together and wished her luck. I don't know if it made her feel any better, but it allowed me to close a

"Obese men and women are equally unhappy in their marriages."

Fiction. All is not equal in marriage between the sexes, at least not when it comes to being overweight and being happy. In one study, obese women were happier with their marriages than other women, whereas obese men had more marital problems. Also, men who gained weight once they were married were more likely to report marital problems than men who lost weight, while married women who gained weight were more likely to be happy compared with other wives who lost weight.

Why the differences? One theory about why obese women are happier with their marriages is that they realize that their "value" in the marriage market is lower because the United States still stigmatizes obesity. As a result, obese women are more likely to be satisfied with their current marital situation and prefer it to potentially seeking a new partner. On the other hand, obese men may be more likely to have marital problems because their wives may pressure them to lose weight, leading to hostility and conflict in their marriages. Also, men may be less likely to accept the negative social view about their body weight than women, who just live with the stigma that carrying extra body fat bestows upon them.

chapter in my life that had brought a lot of pain and fear.

Love and Marriage as a Formerly Obese Man

To say my perspective on relationships, in particular marriage, has changed would be the understatement of the century. I met my wife, Suzy, on the show. I remember when I met her. It was the first day of taping, and we had just arrived at the Ranch. We were all crammed into a fifteen-passenger van, and it was nearly a hundred degrees out. Imagine a van full of obese people sitting out in the sun. "Hot and sweaty" doesn't even begin to describe the discomfort I was feeling.

After a long while, I finally got sick, and I can remember seeing a look of disbelief on Suzy's face. Neither one of us said a word.

As the show progressed on the Ranch, I began to dislike Suzy even more. I couldn't figure out why she was always so happy. I mean, what did she have to be happy about? She was twenty-nine years old, single, and fat. I felt that she should be just as angry as I was. Suzy was different, though. She worked out as hard as anyone else on the Ranch and was a fierce competitor, but when she wasn't working out, she was giggly and seemed to really enjoy being herself. It wasn't until a couple of weeks into the show that I learned that her joy in life came from being a committed Christian and that her reason for

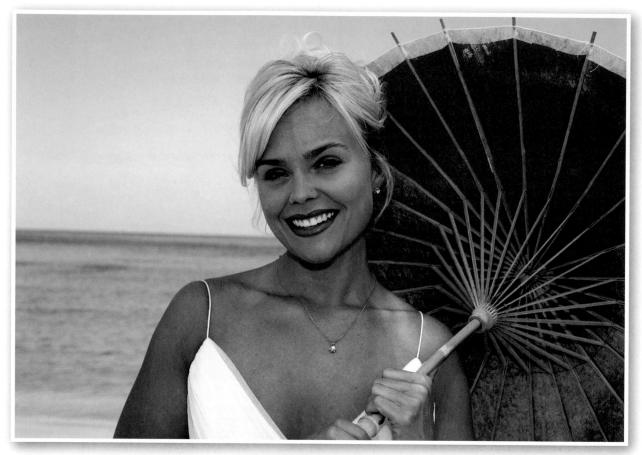

My beautiful bride on our wedding day, photographed by Rebecca Bouck.

being on the show was just to "give it a try." It turns out that Suzy hadn't even watched the first season of the show and only ended up on our season at the last minute. She wasn't even really sure she wanted to do it at all. These things coupled together only frustrated me even more. I was there to win! For her to say that she didn't really know anything about the show just rubbed me the wrong way. Who in his or her right mind wouldn't come on to the show to try to win the $250,000 prize? That's why I was there: I wanted the money.

At the beginning of the show, I had only one really close friend. Mark and I have similar personalities, and we worked well together. After watching the "girls" self-destruct for the first few weeks because of arguing and fighting amongst themselves, we thought we had figured out exactly how to take them all out. One night on the way to the weigh-ins, Suzy turned to Mark and said, "Please send me home," with tears in her eyes. We both looked at each other and grinned because we couldn't believe our good fortune. Someone had just admitted that she really didn't want to be there, and we were about to exploit it.

The girls lost the weigh-in that night and had to pick one of them to send home. Their team had become so disenchanted with each other that they couldn't even come to an agreement on which one of them should get booted out. Consequently, the vote was left

up to the men's team. Mark and I explained to all the guys what we felt was happening on the women's team and how we could really start to dismantle their team. Suzy had become close to one of the girls on her team, and although Suzy was the one who wanted to go home, we figured that by sending her close friend home instead, she would hate it on the Ranch so much that she'd want to quit and ease up on her workouts. We also thought that if she didn't want to be there, it might make the chemistry on the girls' team even worse. Needless to say, that night we voted to send home Suzy's closest ally. We were all smiles when we left the elimination room because we thought our little plan had worked like a charm. The girls were even more divided, and we were going to just sit back and wait to send Suzy packing.

Well, our strategy to rattle Suzy didn't work as we had planned. Rather than sit around and feel sorry for herself, she added even more intensity to her workouts. As it turned out, we never did get the chance to get rid of her because she was never up for possible elimination again after that night. As I watched Suzy work out, she began to earn my respect, whether she cared or not that was about that. I had been a NCAA Division I athlete, and no one was supposed to be able to work out as hard as I did. She was pretty close, and I thought that was cool.

On one episode, we were all supposed to get makeovers. I was not thrilled about this at all. I had long curly hair and had not had a haircut in over two years, and I wanted to keep it. My hair was like a security blanket. I could hide behind it and still delude myself into believing that it made me look thinner. (It didn't.) Long story short, everyone but me got haircuts and dye jobs. They

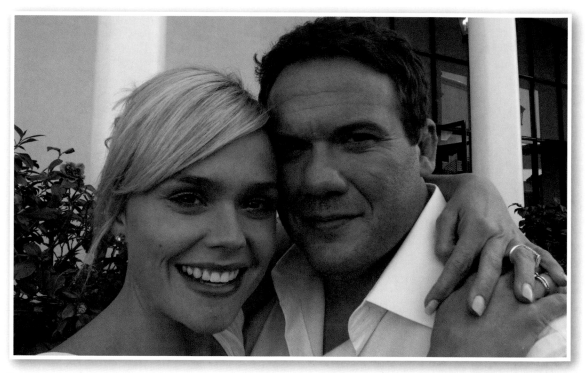

At a Details magazine shoot.

took about a quarter of an inch off my hair and called it done. After the makeovers, we went to a photo shoot for a national magazine. I was still pouting and looked like a big jerk in all the photos.

That night when we got home, I looked around at all of the contestants and noticed how much they had changed in our time on the Ranch. They all looked so good. I felt like I looked exactly the same. The others were all walking around with a new air of confidence and new-found self-respect, and I was feeling (and looking) like the same old angry Matt.

The day after the makeovers, we had a challenge during which we got to see one of our family members for a brief time. My dad said, "You look great, but you still haven't cut that hair, huh?" I didn't think much of it—he had never really liked my long hair anyway—but that night, I started to examine why I still hadn't cut my hair. What it really came down to was that I was afraid to let myself be a new

person. After that realization, I went to talk to one of the producers and asked if there was any way that I could go ahead and get my hair cut off. They said it was a little late, but that they would see what they could do. One night not long afterwards, Suzy came into my room with a set of scissors. Of all people, she was the one who was going to cut my hair. There were two ladies who were hairstylists on the Ranch, and they still picked Suzy. I remember thinking, "I hope she doesn't stab me with those scissors."

A funny thing happened as she began to cut my hair. As each lock fell to the floor, I began to feel different. I felt lighter and happier, like a new person was being released. When Suzy was all done cutting it short, I couldn't believe how great I felt. This annoying woman who squealed when she laughed had allowed me to become a new person right in front of her, and she had helped make it so. I think I might have even given her a hug. From then on, I found myself smiling a lot more and acting like a different person. I also began to view Suzy differently. We spent time together talking and found out that we had a lot in common, including similar ideas and likes and dislikes. At that point, you could say that we were fast becoming friends.

One day toward the end of the show, one of our trainers took us shopping for some new clothes, since none of us had any that still fit. I found myself asking Suzy how all the clothes I tried on looked and what she thought about this and that. Toward the end of the shopping day, I was trying to find new cologne, and the lady behind the counter remarked how nice it was to see a couple having so much fun together. Suzy and I both laughed because of the absurdity of the comment. Us, a couple? No way! Nonetheless, we continued to spend time together—as friends.

Shortly thereafter, we had to leave the Ranch and continue to lose weight at home. We weren't allowed to see each other again until the final weigh-in on *The Biggest Loser* season finale. I had wondered what Suzy would look like, and I was shocked when I saw her on the stage. She was stunning and still had a smile that could light up a room. When the host asked me what I thought about how she looked, I could only stare in disbelief. She looked like a model.

After the finale was over, I had to jet off to New York to make appearances the next morning. Before I left, Suzy came into my dressing room and asked what I was thinking and if I still liked her. I said definitely and that I would talk to her when I got back to L.A. in a couple days for a photo shoot. For the first time, I felt that we could actually become a real couple. I had a lot of fun with her no matter what we were doing, and we just clicked.

In September of the year after the show ended, we got married in Jamaica at the beautiful Grand Lido Resort, with only our immediate family members present. It was truly a fairy-tale wedding. I know without a doubt that when I watched Suzy walk down the path to where we were to become husband and wife, I was watching the most beautiful woman on earth, who was walking to be with me. I found out later that Suzy had written home during the show informing her family that there was "absolutely no husband material" on the show. Who would have thought that Matt and Suzy from *The Biggest Loser* would be exchanging their vows? It just goes to show you that some of the best things in life come when you're not looking for them.

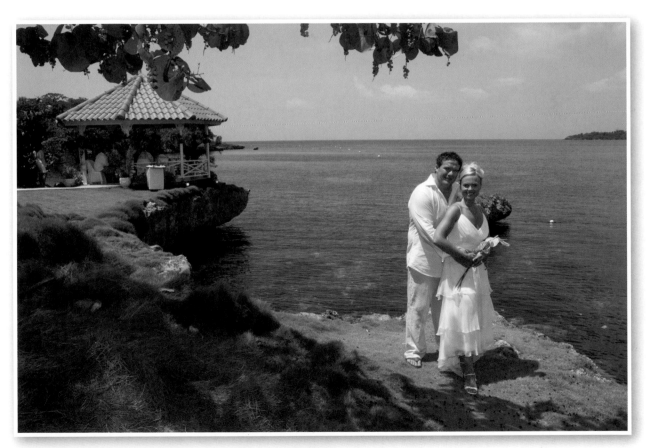

Our wedding at Grand Lido Resort in Jamaica. AMAZING!

My wife and I have an extraordinary relationship. I love being married to her and can't wait to get home at the end of a speaking engagement or after being away from her for any reason—both because of our shared faith and the lessons that I learned on the show. I learned that before I could care for someone else, I had to care for myself. When a person isn't willing to take care of himself, how can he possibly take care of someone else? Before, I had felt that as long as people around me were happy, I myself was happy—not true. I think many of my previous relationships had suffered

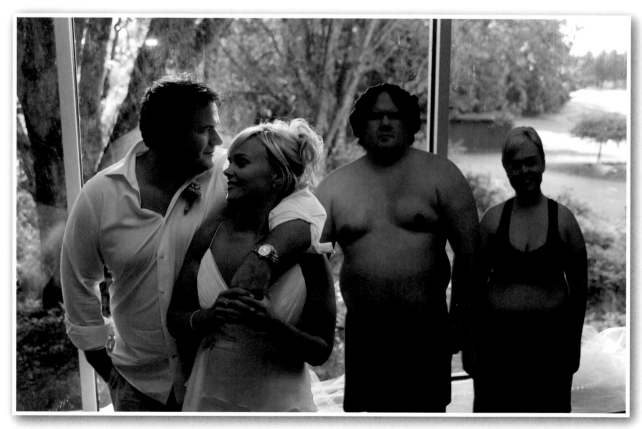

Looking back at where this all started.

because I was looking outside of myself to someone else to increase the happiness in my own life. My wife makes me happy, but it's because I am able to give her back all the happiness that she gives to me; it goes both ways. When I start to feel down, I instinctively start to pull back. My wife, being my helpmate as well, recognizes this and is not afraid to say something, which has helped me a lot.

Dr. Sheri's Tips on Loving Yourself Enough to Be Able to Love Others

- In order to really love someone else, you must first learn how to love and respect yourself, or else your relationship will be based on needs, not mutual respect.
- Carefully choose the messages you give to yourself by employing positive self-talk.
- Change your messages for the better, keeping only positive ones, like "I am loveable."
- Repeat these affirmations daily and often throughout each day.
- Choose to reject negative messages, ones like "I'm too fat for anyone to love" or "I'm a failure because I can't lose weight." ➡

- Take charge and improve your self-image through assertive behaviors, rather than passive ones (e.g., ask questions, gather information, and elicit help from others).

- Positive behaviors create positive feelings, so doing something nice for someone else can help you feel better about yourself.

- Learn how to better accept compliments when you receive them, and give them to other people as well.

- Praise yourself for what you do that is positive each day (such as passing on an extra treat that you knew you didn't need to eat).

- Thank other people and be generous in giving them praise.

- Give yourself a pep talk from time to time (e.g., say to yourself, "I can do this").

- Keep a personal file with all of your affirming notes, cards, or other mementos that you can look through from time to time.

CHAPTER 6

Crying Is Not Just for Sissies

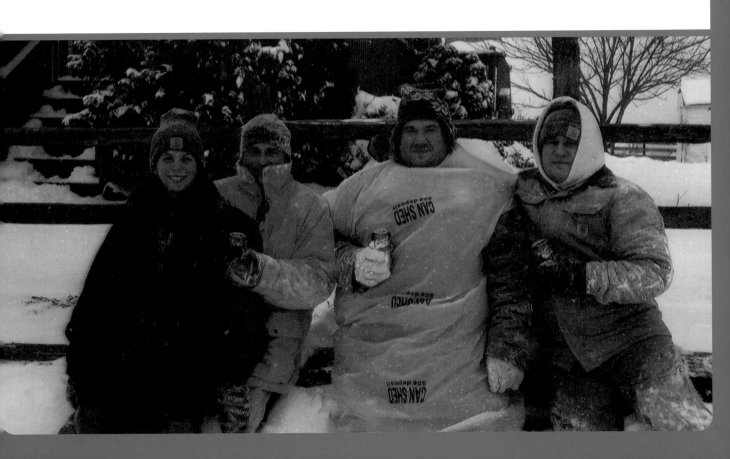

I have always been a pretty emotional guy, but being on *The Biggest Loser* seemed to bring my emotions to a whole new level. One of the criticisms of the show and of me in particular was that the emotion being shown on nearly every episode appeared staged. It wasn't. I am not an actor, and there was enough other drama going on that was way more exciting than my shedding tears.

The fact of the matter is that I was at a very difficult point in my life, and to say that being on the show and battling my weight were easy emotionally would be like saying that Dan Gable was just a mediocre, small-time wrestling coach—that is, totally off base. It was more like the wildest roller coaster you can think of, as far as my emotions went. I had a lot to go through to sort out my emotions, and I learned that it was better to let them bubble to the surface and deal with them than to let them stay buried, where they only added to the pool of pain that remained trapped inside of me for many years.

Taking a Good Look at Yourself Can Be Painful

I had a lot going on during the show, both emotionally and physically. There was no drinking allowed at the Ranch during our season, so I had to stop my alcohol intake cold turkey. For a guy who drank as much as I did, this was a major shock to my system. I had used alcohol to mask many of my hurts, to celebrate, to relax, and to entertain. Alcohol had been a big part of my life for many years, and then suddenly it was completely gone.

For the first time in my life I felt truly alone. When at home, I was almost always around people, which allowed me to not think about what was going on in my head. When I was alone with my thoughts at the Ranch, I began to think back over the course of my life, and I was more than a little sad. One of the first things that caused me to feel enough of the hurt inside of me to cry on national TV was how I treated my little brother. When we were growing up, my brother was always a chubby kid. As I got older, I made fun of him and called him names like "big 'un" and other less than flattering names. When we competed against each other in wrestling practice, I was always a little mean or said negative things that I didn't need to. My brother marched to his own drum, and because it didn't sound like mine, I made it tough on him. It wasn't until I became obese myself and had to endure similar experiences that I somewhat understood how tough it must have been for him. I was only obese for a few years, but I made fun of my brother and his weight for at least eighteen years.

When I had time on the Ranch to reflect on my behavior toward Timmy, I felt genuine remorse. You know, I can't remember how many gold medals I won over the years, but I can remember, to the word, comments that people made about my weight and exactly who said what. Forget the saying "Sticks and stones may break my bones,

but names will never hurt me." The truth is that words can hurt and leave scars as deep as from any knife. The pain can last for a lifetime. Realizing that I had caused my bother that kind of hurt made me realize that I had not always been a nice person.

Overweight people are the only remaining group in our country that it is somewhat socially acceptable to make fun of. Think about it: if you tell a fat joke or make a snide comment about someone who is overweight, people laugh. Compare that with the fact that if you make a racial slur, you can plan on being reprimanded on the spot; if you do it at a place of employment, more than likely you will be fired. Making fun of or being intolerant of someone's sexuality is now completely taboo. My point is that people have feelings, and overweight people deserve to be treated with respect and decency.

The words of others can cause pain beyond our comprehension. Having been on the receiving end, as well as the one doling

The Effect of Food on Your Mood

How many times have you found yourself eating out of boredom or because of stress, social pressure, or other reasons? Eating certain foods elicits the release of various brain hormones that can actually soothe anxiety and depression, but only up to a point. Overindulging in foods like chocolate (even if it's the healthier dark type) to enhance your mood can later leave you feeling guilty and depressed over the weight you may have gained or from the elevations in blood glucose levels that result from your binge. Moreover, emotional eating can result in longer-term issues and a dysfunctional relationship with food.

Research has also shown that eating sugar and consuming caffeine to alter your mood at best gives you a temporary emotional "high," which will more often than not be followed by a "crash." If you're looking for an emotional pick-me-up from food, some options may have a more positive long-term effect. Among the better choices are foods high in omega-3 fatty acids (e.g., fish and many nuts), which are also good for the health of your cardiovascular system. Healthy carbohydrates like those found in whole fruits, replete with fiber, vitamins and minerals, and phytonutrients, also have a soothing effect—in moderation, of course. For the sake of your emotional health, try to avoid bingeing on highly refined carbohydrates. Also focus on taking in enough of the B vitamins, particularly thiamin, folate, niacin, B6, and B12, which are found in abundance in high-fiber carbohydrate foods like legumes and whole grains. Drinking plenty of water or other non-caloric, non-caffeinated fluids also helps, as does making sure that you eat a healthy breakfast every morning.

out hurtful words in the past, has given me a unique perspective. Today I am glad that I had to go through those experiences. It makes me aware of how my actions can affect others, whether I know them personally or not. I shed many tears on the show from just thinking about the way I treated others, especially my brother, and reflecting on those actions.

Go Ahead and Cry

Prior to going to the Ranch, I believed that I had already done a good job of dealing with my past, specifically my time at the University of Iowa as both a student and an athlete. As I reflected on the things that had gotten me to the Ranch, my wrestling career kept moving to the front. When I was working hard and having a considerable amount of success, I felt good. I was used to succeeding. When I quit wrestling, I didn't know what to do with myself. I had prided myself on being a hard worker and now for the first time that I could recall, I was doing nothing. To make myself feel better I reasoned that I had spent a good portion of my life wrestling and that I deserved a break. I could take some time, relax, and think about my future.

I took some time to relax—several years in fact—but I didn't think much about my future. In fact, I found myself thinking about my past way more. I thought about how I had been given a scholarship to compete for the best wrestling team in the country with the greatest coaching staff in the history of college wrestling. I thought about how I had urinated that opportunity right down my leg. I thought about how in doing so, I had let down my mom, my dad, my friends, my coaches, and even the people in the town I grew up in. I spent so much time thinking about my past that I got stuck living there.

Believe it or not, I had gotten so used to living in my past that when I got to the Ranch, I actually believed that I was still a Hawkeye wrestler—at least physically. I thought I was in the kind of shape I was in when I was running steps and wrestling every day and that all I needed to do was lose a little weight. When I finally accepted the fact that I was no longer a college athlete and was, in fact, an obese, ex-wrestler college dropout, I was devastated. When you discover that everything you believed to be true about yourself is not the truth, you may find yourself wanting to cry. That's what I did.

I think the majority of my tears, however, resulted from the harsh realization that all was not right with me, particularly my physical health. When I heard the words pre-diabetic and hypertensive, I was scared. Only twenty-nine years old, I was shocked by the thought of having to take medications the rest of my life for my health problems. What's more, I began to think that at any moment during a workout, I could possibly drop dead of a heart attack. Fear played yet another big role in my shedding of tears.

"If you're in a bad mood, there is nothing you can do to get out of it."

Fiction. While it is generally healthier not to run away from your feelings and to be able to feel and express them instead, it's not helpful to wallow in self-pity or depression. It's important for your overall emotional health not to get stuck in painful or negative emotions that can lower your self-esteem, cause depression, or lead to negative behaviors like stress eating or an inability to motivate yourself to exercise. For some reason, any emotion or thought that we experience for more than fifteen seconds starts to link to all the other times we felt that way, so focusing on something painful or unpleasant for too long becomes magnified by your similar previous experiences. Too many negative emotions can overwhelm you and reinforce the way you're currently feeling (or make you feel worse).

When you're in a bad mood, you need to be able to shift into a more positive one—in essence, turning that frown upside down into a smile instead. (Don't you hate it when someone says that to you when you're in a bad mood, though?) You do have the power to do this; all it takes is a little practice. It's not something you were likely ever taught, but you can learn how to do it all the same.

Real Men Don't Cry? Who Says?

I could write an entire book about the reasons why I was so emotional on the show; however, it would probably take an army of psychiatrists and counselors to get through all the layers. It's a little like when, in the movie *Shrek,* Shrek explains to Donkey that ogres have layers, and in order to really know an ogre, you have to peel back all of them. The great thing about getting to the bottom of all the layers in humans is that then you can begin to heal. What it all boils down to is that I was an emotional wreck because I had convinced myself that I had lost all of my

opportunities to be successful in athletics and in my life.

The amazing thing about all the crying that took place was that I never even once felt a little bit embarrassed about it. I was healing and letting go of years' worth of frustration and disappointment. With each tear I shed, I was moving further away from my old self and pressing on toward a new and better life. I had bottled up years of hurt that were released through all of those tears.

Many men get uneasy when they see another guy cry. They view crying as a sign of weakness and will poke fun at someone for showing his emotions. In my mind, I would rather see guys shed a few tears than go out and hurt themselves or someone else in order to let off some steam. We are conditioned as men to bottle up our feelings and just suck it up. One of the most frustrating examples of this occurs nearly every Saturday during the winter at little kids' wrestling tournaments across the country. Though most parents are supportive of their kids at these events, I have seen little wrestlers come off the mat crying after losing a match, only to be greeted by a yelling dad who is telling them how disappointed he is in his son. At that young age, the little kid is learning that it is better not to show how he feels about losing after trying his hardest. Unfortunately, many kids get off easier by throwing a tantrum after losing than they do for letting a few tears fall. It is little wonder that most grown men have a tough time showing emotions.

Is crying a sign of weakness? I honestly don't think so, not just because I do it, but because every man has done it at least once in his life, no matter how tough he is. I am a big fan of the UFC, or mixed martial arts. The men and women who participate in that sport are well versed not only in wrestling, but also in boxing, jiu-jitsu, judo, and other various martial arts. These people train in a manner that most of us can't even begin to fathom. Many cry when they lose, and others cry when they win. I can't even imagine some Joe off the street walking up to one of those fighters after a loss and making fun of him for crying. Joe would probably get knocked out if he did.

When people put their heart and soul into a task, regardless of what it is, some emotions will go along with that dedication. That emotion is a good thing; in fact, it may be the very thing that keeps them motivated when it gets nasty along the way. If tears come, fine; if they don't, that's okay as well. I personally don't think anyone has the right to belittle someone for showing emotions, and I'm glad to see men, in particular, be strong enough to let their true feelings show.

On that note, I'd like to say this: go ahead and cry … or don't. Just have a healthy outlet for your emotions and feelings. Unlike when I was on the show, I now deal with my emotions by openly communicating with my wife and by exercising, as well as using visualization techniques. Today I feel like I am well adjusted and well equipped to deal with my emotions, whether I cry or not.

Fact or Fiction?

"The release of endorphins is good for your mood and your physical health."

Fact. One of the purported emotional benefits of exercise is related to the release of brain hormones called endorphins. These mood-enhancing hormones bind to your brain's natural receptors and are responsible for the so-called runner's high, which is a feeling of euphoria after you have been exercising for a while. Those of us who don't run call it our second wind, which is when we start feeling good enough to keep on exercising. Some people are positively addicted to this release of endorphins and need to get their daily dose.

There is another reason why exercise-induced endorphin release is so good for you: endorphins may actually improve your body's insulin action, thereby reversing or decreasing the insulin resistance that leads to pre-diabetes or type 2 diabetes, both of which are more common if you're overweight or obese. It is now thought that endorphin release may be a major mechanism in enhanced insulin sensitivity attributable to moderate exercise training. Go for maximum endorphins on a daily basis, and as a side benefit, you will be less depressed and anxious and enjoy a greatly improved mood.

The Three Most Important Things I Learned About Myself on the Show

Let me tell you a little about the most important things I learned about myself on the show. Prior to going on it, I thought I knew who I was. In my mind, I was the happy, fat guy that people liked to be around, so that is who I became. I also thought that I was perfectly happy being that guy. My time on the show made me realize that I wasn't happy at all with either my mental or physical state.

I think the most important thing I learned was that I was directly responsible for my own position in life. I had chosen how I was going to live, and I was responsible for the consequences. Until about halfway through the show, I was waiting to fail. Failure had become a part of my mindset, and I was constantly looking over my shoulder with the expectation that things from my past would catch up with me once again and throw a wrench, so to speak, in my current success. I finally understood that my past failures and pain no longer had to affect my present and future. Blaming others for my failures had allowed me to continue making the same mistakes while repeatedly getting the same results.

Every individual is full of potential, but most simply don't know how to fulfill it. In that respect, I was no different. From the time I was a little boy, I had always heard people remark about how much potential and talent I had if I would just apply my-self. I always seemed to get by and never really had to apply myself. It was that kind of attitude that led me into being an obese person on a reality TV show: a big loser.

The second lesson I took away from the Ranch is that it is never too late to change. When the show started, the only change I intended to make was to my body weight. I believed that I was happy and that if only my weight were under control, I would be a brand-new man. The fact of the matter

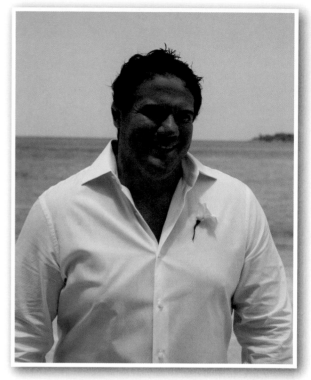

Me on my wedding day.

is that if I hadn't taken the steps to change myself on the inside, my physical changes would have been pretty meaningless.

Have you ever seen a really crappy look-ing old car driving down the road? I'm talk-ing about an obviously being-restored car: flat gray, still dented, maybe a little rusted. It just looks like a mess. As the car goes past, you hear it. Whether you know anything about cars or not, you can tell that this car is obviously not running very well. It is hitting on all cylinders, as they say. The person driving that car knows something very important: it doesn't really matter what the car looks like on the outside if it is running well. With a little cosmetic work and a fresh coat of paint, that car will look great. However, without repairs to the inside of the car (for example, the motor), it doesn't matter how good the rest of the vehicle looks because it will just be a pile of junk in the driveway.

What I'm getting at is this: people who restore classic cars begin with the inside and work their way out. They rebuild the motor, then move to the interior of the car, and eventually work on the outside of the vehicle. When they are done, they can be sure they did a good restoration because they took the right steps. Even though at times the job was probably tedious, the end result was worth all the hours that they invested.

In essence, I learned that I needed an overhaul. Even though I was nearly thirty and was pretty set in my ways, I understood I needed to change, and that the change had to come from the inside out in order to last. Seeing the physical change was easy—there were cameras that documented my every lost pound—but it was a lot harder to see what was going on inside. I have said from the beginning of this journey that the hardest part of losing weight is keeping it off. The reason it is so difficult is because many of us maintain our old ways of thinking, even after we lose weight. We fail to realize that the destructive thoughts we had when we were obese will continue to be destructive when we are healthy—if we don't work on changing them.

Physical change starts with moving your body. Emotional improvements leading to lasting change start with working your mind. Replacing negative and self-destructive thoughts with positive and productive ones will allow you to become a new and improved individual. I finally understood that I couldn't move forward with my new life if I was going to try and hold on to old habits and thoughts. The reason that I had gotten to the point of despair was because I was afraid to commit to change. I knew that if I really wanted it, I would have to give up some of the very things that had provided comfort for so long, namely drinking and overeating.

So, when you decide to commit to changing your ways, you have to start from the inside out. Even though it is hard work, it is worth it. The really great thing about approaching change in this way is that, just like that old car, with the right care and skill, regardless of how bad the original damage was, a worn-out, damaged person can successfully be healed from the inside out and restored to a new and better life.

The third and perhaps most enlightening lesson that came from being on the show is the understanding that being healthy is going to be a lifelong journey. I have lost and gained hundreds of pounds over the years, failing to realize that it doesn't have to be an endless cycle. I had always lost weight and dieted with the idea that after I reached my goal, I could start eating however I wanted to again. In essence, my reward for getting healthy had always been to revert back to being unhealthy by rewarding myself with food or a night out. As I mentioned, I made changes so that I wouldn't have to change. By making just enough of a temporary change to feel like I was on track, I could easily go back to my old ways without feeling bad or like it was all a waste of time.

I have since found out that it doesn't matter how hard you worked in the past or how much weight you have lost; regardless, being healthy is a daily exercise, literally. My wife and I decided even before we got married that we were determined to live healthy, active lives. Making that commitment requires dedication—to healthy eating, to working out and doing something physical on a daily basis, to being honest with each

"Learning how to relax can help you deal with life's daily problems more effectively."

Fact. A good idea is to use the time while you exercise to simultaneously work on your emotional health through relaxation techniques. Specifically, learn to optimize your mental and physical health by following the RIB principle: "R" for relaxation, "I" for imagination, and "B" for breathing. Try to relax while you are exercising; let your troubles flow out of your body; punch the air with your fists to release your anger or anxiety; and consciously try to relax the tense muscles in your body. Also, use your imagination to visualize more blood flowing to parts of your body that need it, like your heart and muscles. Finally, take slow, deep, and steady breaths and release them slowly as well. Don't do this during heavy aerobic exercise, however; use the time during your warm-up and cool-down periods instead for best results. At any time during a workout, take deeper breaths if you are feeling winded, because more oxygen is brought into your body during a deep breath than a shallow one. That fact may be a large part of why deep, slow breathing has such a relaxing, calming effect.

other about our goals and aspirations, and to using the skills we have learned for the rest of our lives.

I have struggled with binge eating since I was young. During a binge, I would eat a large pizza by myself and still not feel full. If I binged at a buffet, I would typically eat until I physically could not fit one more bite in my stomach. Many times I would even vomit in the parking lot from being too full. In the movie *Super Size Me*, you saw the guy making the documentary do the same thing after stuffing himself too full of McDonald's food.

My binges were usually emotionally triggered. If I was having a bad day, I would plan where I was going to eat and what. If it was Chinese food, I knew exactly where the buffet was located. Sometimes I would wake up in the middle of night from a sound sleep, get in the car, drive to a late-night taco place, and order ten tacos at the drive-through. Then I'd eat them all before I got home, which was less than a mile away. In my mind, if I ate really fast, it didn't count. That's how bad my urges were—bad enough for me to get out of bed in the middle of the night and drive so I could stuff myself.

Another ritual that I had was that every Sunday I would go to the restaurant and order the Chinese dinner for four. My thought process was that I would eat the leftovers throughout the week. That is what I told myself, anyway. But I knew I was about to destroy a dinner that should have fed three others along with me. I share these details because now I have to be prepared for my former habits to creep back at any time, and being aware of them is the only way to stop them from returning. In order for me to live a healthy life and to move forward, I need to understand my triggers and have a plan ready to implement immediately when those old thoughts start resurfacing.

My triggers are the same as for many others who suffer from obesity: feeling happy or sad, reaching a big goal or missing one, having family in town to visit, or celebrating an occasion. Any of those—pretty much anything—can trigger my old thought process. How do I avoid giving in? The answer is simply that I have a plan to combat it. My house is a safe zone. My wife and I have agreed that we won't bring things into our home that won't help us to achieve our goals. If I am out and about and can fight off the particular urge that I have and get home, more than likely it will dissipate.

Another strategy is to use visualization techniques. I know exactly how I feel when I give into a binge. During the episode I am numb, and all I think about is what I am going to eat next. After the episode, I feel physically ill and sad. Now when I feel a binge coming on, I recall the feelings I have had in the past and determine if it is going to be worth feeling that way right now. It usually isn't. If visualization doesn't work, I call my wife. I tell her exactly what I am about to do, and she asks me point blank what is going on and if bingeing will actually help. By verbalizing my feelings, I am better able to deal with the emotions that can trigger binges.

There are still times when I want to binge, but I have practiced reprogramming my thoughts and having backup plans. I have the support of my wife and know that the feelings I am experiencing are temporary and can be overcome. By understanding that this is a battle I will face the rest of my life, I can prepare myself for the ups and downs and hopefully encounter fewer downs. I'm not afraid of living my life, because I am now confident that I am armed with all the emotional and physical tools that I need to succeed.

Dr. Sheri's Tips for Turning That Frown Upside Down (and Relieving Stress)

- Find a way to laugh, even if it's just at a silly joke, a ridiculous situation, or someone's inane antics.

- Take a walk and temporarily get out of the environment that you're in (i.e., go outside if you're inside or vice versa).

- Change your body posture, take some deep breaths; relax your shoulders, lean back in your chair, and let all the stress go.

- Do something physical that requires concentration, such as balancing on one leg with your other leg extended and your arms up; if that's too easy, close your eyes and try to do it.

- Change your perspective by looking for the positive in every situation or person; once you get used to looking for it, you'll find it more easily each time.

- Reframe your thoughts, especially if they're negative; stop saying things like "I can't," "I shouldn't," and "I'll never," and change them into positives instead (like "I can").

- Close your eyes and think of a person who loves you; concentrate hard, and really feel the love for thirty seconds or more.

- Reach out to a friend who you can talk to when your emotions are piling up on you.
- Smell something pleasant that you like, like bread baking, fresh air, or flowers; your sense of smell is a powerful tool for controlling your emotions.

CHAPTER 7

Just Do It

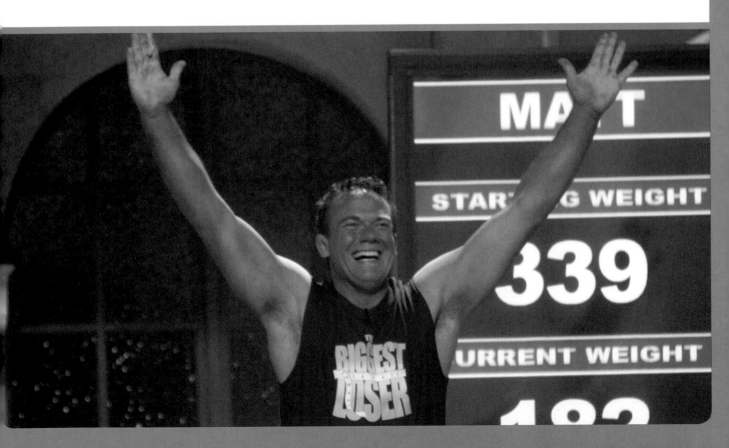

You've all heard the Nike brand motto, "Just do it." Sometimes that's just what you have to keep saying to yourself. It's not always that easy, I know! Willpower is a funny thing. You may have the best of intentions, and then something waylays your plans. You do have some control over your attitudes and your outlook on life, and it's those emotional aspects of losing weight that I want to talk to you about now. You've got to find the motivation to stick with your plan to lose weight, even if it's finding out that you have some health problems that you're "too young" to have. In this chapter, I'm going to tell you what worked best for me.

Visualize Your Successes

Why do people lose weight only to gain it all back, if not more? I myself have lost hundreds of pounds over my lifetime. I even gained a little after being on national television, though I lost it again before it got out of hand. It wasn't until I started with my personal trainer, PJ Glassey, at the X Gym in Seattle, Washington, that I learned about the importance of the mental and emotional aspects of weight maintenance. As an athlete, I certainly understood the importance of mental preparation; I was able to implement mental toughness into not only my wrestling competitions, but also my training. However, I had never associated it with staying in shape when it came to losing weight and keeping it off.

Whether you are an athlete or not, you have probably heard the phrase, "You will only perform as well as you practice." Tiger Woods doesn't sit around all week doing nothing and then go out and win every tournament he plays. Undoubtedly, he spends hours getting prepared and practicing to stay on top of his game. Part of being a great athlete is having the ability to visualize the outcome of the event you are training for. I have yet to encounter an elite athlete who visualizes failing at an event. Since they don't see failure as an option, the best mentally prepared athletes often win and succeed, even when things get tough, even if they're not necessarily the most naturally gifted competitor.

Many times the best athletes have simply worked and prepared harder than everyone else. The difference between average athletes and the great ones is that the great athletes have gone over every possible scenario in their minds before they begin competing. They visualize what it will be like when they win, including the details of what it's like to compete in the arena—what it will smell and sound like—and how it will feel to be crowned the champion. They have spent hours visualizing and mentally practicing for success.

What does all this have to do with trying to lose weight and successfully keeping it off? Everything! In order to be successful, we need to be willing to visualize ourselves as successful. I can't count how many people I have heard say to me, "I have tried everything, but nothing works for me." These people are starting with a self-defeating attitude, certain that they will fail before they even begin. And the real kicker is that whether they're conscious of it or not, they will actually do everything they can to fail.

For several years after I left the University of Iowa, I would start out with a goal in mind, only to fall short. I would get this close to succeeding, and then I would sabotage myself and set myself up to fail. I did this over and over, until I began to feel like I didn't deserve to have success of any kind in my life—not in weight loss, my career, or my relationships. With this type of thinking, it's not hard to figure out how I eventually became angry and bitter. I had essentially convinced myself that I was a failure and that nothing I did was ever right.

This nonproductive line of thought followed me right into my approach to diet and exercise. I felt like my best years were behind me and that I had nothing to look forward to, so why even try? The more I felt sorry for myself, the worse off I became. Although I knew I was uncomfortable in my own skin, I let myself believe that the lifestyle that I was living was the life—the only life—for me, my destiny. The funny thing about feeling sorry for myself was that the worse I felt, the more self-destructive my behavior became. Looking back on it now, I think I was almost trying to see how bad I could make it for myself. By making my situation appear abysmal, I provided a ready-made excuse for living like I was.

When I began the show and my ensuing journey to get healthy, I found myself following this same pattern: I still tried to make things difficult for myself. Although I knew I could win, I was afraid of what might happen if I did. On more than one occasion, I looked for reasons why I should leave the show or cause myself to be sent home. Finally, it took some outside events to get me off of this pathway and on the road to success.

"I Never Had You Pegged as a Quitter"

My turning point came after a series of events that made me question everything. During my time on the Ranch, I had learned that the company I had been working for had been bought out and that I probably wouldn't have a job anymore when I got home. Right after that, I went out for a hike and got completely covered in poison ivy. Then I found out that my uncle had just died of a heart attack. Needless to say, after all that I was feeling pretty sorry for myself.

To compound everything, that week's challenge at the Ranch involved the opportunity to see family members. My reward, if I were to win the challenge, was to spend some time with my dad, who had just lost his brother. Being able to comfort my dad in person would have been especially important for me, since I was not able to leave the Ranch to go to my uncle's funeral. The challenge consisted of riding a bike with

"It's unusual for your body weight to fluctuate during the day."

Fiction. Actually, it would be unusual for your weight *not* to change during the day. Your daily weight fluctuations have more to do with changes in your water content than anything else. The human body is usually about 60 percent water. If you get dehydrated, you'll weigh less, until you drink enough to replace the fluid. Conversely, if you drink and eat a lot, your weight will be higher for a while until your body has processed it and gotten rid of the extra water and roughage. Your weight can also go up following a day when you've feasted well (like Thanksgiving) and not done much exercise, due to storing glycogen in your muscles (along with extra water). Even if you weigh five pounds more, or less, from one day to the next, you can't assume the weight gain, or loss, is permanent. If you monitor your body weight closely, then be sensible and measure it at the same time each day, preferably first thing in the morning.

a compartment that we pulled behind the bike for our family member (like one of those carriers for kids) up a hill. The winner was allowed to spend the evening with his or her chosen relative. I started out fast, but died out toward the end and finished second. I threw a little tantrum because I was also feeling sorry for myself for not getting to spend time with my dad.

As I was walking up to return to the house where we were all staying, I saw one of the show's producers. I pulled him aside and informed him that I was going to throw the next weigh-in and get myself sent home. He listened to all that I had to say and all the reasons I gave for wanting to leave, and then he replied, "I never had you pegged for a quitter." I had just poured out my soul looking for someone to feel sorry for me, and that was all I was going to get as a response? I figured he should at least have said something to make me want to stay.

Looking back, I'm glad he didn't try to make me feel all warm and fuzzy about my decision to leave. I went up to my room and began to think about what that producer had said. He was right: leaving the show then would have been quitting. Sure, I had good reasons for wanting to go home, but when it came right down to it, I would have been the quitter the producer was talking about. As I sat there, I began to think back over the past several years of my life and the decisions I had made that put me where I was prior to coming on the show. I thought about my choices and how I had arrived at this place where it seemed better to give up than to stick it out and fight.

The longer I sat there, the more my mind returned to the day I left the University of Iowa and walked away from the sport of wrestling. Revisiting that moment made me realize that the majority of my problems stemmed from that decision alone, probably directly because of it. Up until that point, I can't remember having quit anything in my life. No matter how tough things were or how bad I hated doing something, I had stuck it out. Once I made the decision to quit the first time in college, it got easier and easier to give up on other things. Although it started with school and wrestling, it carried over to my jobs, relationships, and anything else that required work. I knew that I had really hit bottom when I finally quit on myself.

Why Do People Lose Their Motivation to Succeed?

Why do people quit? I'm sure there are all sorts of different reasons, but I can tell you why I did. Quitting allowed me not to have to take responsibility for my actions. I quit wrestling because I was always getting hurt. I quit jobs because I didn't like the work. In relationships, I convinced myself that they didn't work out because of her "issues," not mine. Failure was never my fault, and I always had good reasons to justify my actions. After all, no one ever questioned me about the choices I made. How could

they? I obviously had it much worse than anybody else. I deserved to quit.

There I sat at the Ranch, knowing I had a very good shot at winning the show and realizing that I was about to throw in the towel—yet again. I was almost to the point of convincing myself that I deserved to leave and that no one would blame me, especially after the week I had just had. It had come to this, a moment that I had faced over and over for the past six years of my life. I had to choose to either stick it out or pack it up. Prior to the show it would have been an easy decision: I would have left. This time, however, was different. In my time on the show, I had gotten glimpses of the guy who would never give up, the old me as I used to be years before. I remembered how it felt to overcome and end up better, stronger, and more confident that I had been before.

That moment was truly a life-changing one because I was faced with two choices and a decision to make. Choice 1: My life could forever change for the better if I would just

It May Take More than Willpower Alone

Recent research in health and behavioral sciences indicates that willpower alone may not be enough to motivate many people to lose weight, exercise more, and maintain better health habits. Apparently, the physiology of your body, your subconscious mind, and the environment also play strong roles in determining whether your willpower will be enough to prevail.

As for your body's physiology, obesity research shows that once you gain weight, your body works hard to maintain it. With evolution in mind, the feast-or-famine days of our ancestors meant that you had to eat as much as you could when food was plentiful; during the frequent famine times, your body was able to slow down its metabolism and survive on stored body fat. It worked well in those times, but not in our time, when calories are cheap and plentiful most of the time. Fat storage is also affected by a variety of hormones that stimulate weight regain that are released when you lose weight.

As for the power of the mind, why do people oftentimes make stupid choices, even when faced by a host of logical reasons to make the right one? Apparently, it's because the emotional side of your brain has a lot of sway over your behavior; your emotions often override the rational side of your mind and the more logical course of action. This is especially true when it comes to long-term benefits (such as doing exercise for better health down the road) versus short-term unpleasantness (like the physical challenges of doing a hard workout). Emotions like fear or pleasure thwart good choices by changing what you do with your cognitive brain. Chances are, unless you have bad health now that will improve rapidly due to a change in your habits, short-term pleasure will win out over the promise of health benefits down the road.

The environment around you plays a strong role as well. Americans are bombarded with a host of quick, easy, and affordable food options that are also unhealthy. We've come to expect all-you-can-eat buffets, large servings in restaurants, and tasty food enhanced with extra fat, salt, and sugar. How much you eat may even be controlled by your subconscious mind and affected by the environment. For example, when researchers rigged certain soup bowls at a dining table to secretly refill, the people eating from the bottomless bowls ate 73 percent more soup than their meal mates. (Hey, there's still soup ➡

left in your bowl, so why should you stop eating?) It has also been shown that people eat more when serving themselves from larger containers, even if they're told that fact up front. However, leaving all of the emptied plates on the table at a buffet helps decrease how much people eat, while bussing the plates away immediately removes the visual cue that you may have had enough.

Finally, what works best may also differ with how you grew up. For example, to motivate men from lower socioeconomic backgrounds to lose weight, the focus should probably not be on the benefits of leanness and good health, but rather on something that they value more: how losing weight can increase their effectiveness and performance in their jobs (and possibly their earnings).

So when it comes down to it, to be successful at weight loss or any other lifestyle change, you may need specific behavioral skills and an environment conducive to healthy choices, along with the confidence to change your bad habits. Experts recommend manipulating the environment to limit the bad choices and make the good ones available, even by doing simple things like using smaller plates to help you eat less. There's no magic bullet that works for everyone, but some strategies are helpful to many. Set clear, specific goals that are realistic, such as deciding to not buy snacks out of vending machines, as a specific approach to "eating better," or walking thirty minutes a day to "exercise more." Build your confidence, surround yourself with like-minded people, and get plenty of sleep to keep your emotional stress levels manageable and your willpower functioning optimally.

choose to continue to get healthy and win the $250,000 prize, which would pay off every debt I had. Choice 2: I could walk away from the show, let everything stay the same, and let my life continue as it had for the previous several years. With the latter choice, I could have wallowed in self-pity and told everyone how I had been on TV and really should have won, but everything was against me (again). Unlike other times, I made a conscious choice not to be a quitter ... and it paid off! By not giving up that night, I learned that deep down I still had that fighting spirit. I just had to find it again.

Looking back, I realize that I wasn't nearly as afraid of being a quitter as I was of being a success. Since that moment, I have come to believe that many other people are also more afraid of success than they are of failure. The reason I was afraid of coming out on top wasn't because I didn't know how; rather, it was because I knew I was going to have to make some serious changes in my life. I had grown comfortable with being lazy and mediocre. If I were to succeed at this challenge, people would start expecting more out of me. I would expect more out of me, too. To someone used to giving up, realizing that I was making a decision with such ramifications for my whole life was a frightening prospect.

All of this brings me to this point: if you want to be successful at anything, you can't give up. It doesn't matter how many times you have quit in the past. If you truly want to break the cycle, you have to stop being afraid of becoming a success.

When Your Health Is Suffering . . .

I briefly mentioned the health problems that I was having before losing weight, but let me give you a little more detail about how bad they were and how I turned it all around with a better lifestyle. Before I left to be on *The Biggest Loser*, I thought I was in pretty good shape in spite of my weight. Even though I hadn't been to a doctor in years, I thought I was relatively healthy. After all, I was only twenty-nine, and I woke up every morning. I was healthy since I wasn't dead. My logic, although flawed, stemmed from the fact that

all of my grandparents were still alive, my great-grandma on my dad's side lived to be 104, and both of my great-grandparents on my mom's side lived long lives.

In my mind I thought I was invincible, and I lived life exactly that way. I know most guys think that they'll stay young and healthy forever when they're that age, but I wasn't even healthy, due to my lifestyle. I spent the majority of time drinking and eating with friends, but I have never blamed any of them or anyone else for the self-destructive pattern I was in. When I say I spent my time drinking, I mean *really* drinking. My favorite drink was called a rum and rum. The name indicates what was in it. I would take a bottle of Captain Morgan rum and a bottle of Malibu rum, mix them together, and then drink it until I was literally numb. I can't even begin to count the number of times I woke up with very little to no recollection of the prior night's activities. I could write a whole book with the stories I remember (and some that I have

Realistic, Expert Recommendations for Weight Loss and Maintenance

- Aim for an initial weight loss goal of 10 percent of your body weight (e.g., 30 pounds if you weigh 300 pounds).

- Only attempt further weight loss after you're successful and if you still need or want to lose more.

- Follow a diet that creates a deficit of 500 to 1,000 calories per day to lose one to two pounds per week (after the first two weeks).

- Just lowering your fat intake without also eating fewer calories won't be enough to lose weight, but taking in less dietary fat and carbohydrates can help reduce calories.

- Include daily physical activity of various types as an integral part of losing weight and keeping it off.

- Engage in moderate physical activity for at least thirty to forty five minutes three to five days a week to start.

- Accumulate thirty minutes or more of moderate-intensity physical activity on most, and preferably all, days of the week over the long haul. ➡

- Don't just diet; rather combine a reduced calorie intake with increased physical activity to lose bad abdominal fat, retain muscle, and increase your fitness level all at once.
- Permanently change some of the behaviors that caused your weight gain in order to succeed at weight loss and weight maintenance over time.
- If you have lost weight, make a lifelong change in your diet, physical activity, and behaviors to keep it off.
- Focus on weight maintenance after your initial six months of weight loss.
- If you use weight loss drugs, don't take them for longer than a year.

heard from my friends) about my drinking days, but let's just suffice it to say that my biggest health problem prior to being on the show was due to excessive drinking.

I was the type of drinker who drank to get drunk, and the drunker I got, the more I would eat. I remember going on Thursday nights to a bar where you could have all the chicken wings you could eat for two, yes, *two* dollars, and I remember how we got upset when they raised the price to three dollars. I made a bet with my buddies one night that I could eat one hundred wings. I got to eighty-nine before I couldn't stuff any more in my fat face. The reason I share this particular story is because I couldn't figure out why

I suffered from such severe heartburn. Well, drinking straight rum and eating hot wings can't be all that good for one's innards.

My heartburn was so bad that I had to sleep sitting up to alleviate the intense pain that I experienced on a nightly basis. One night I woke up because I thought I had vomited and was drowning. My chest was burning and the sensation went up all the way through my nostrils. I sat up on the side of the bed trying to catch my breath … but I couldn't. I seriously thought that I was having a heart attack. I drove myself to the emergency room, where they explained to me that the acid in my stomach had backed up and was causing the burning. Logic would dictate that after an event like that, I would have made some changes in my eating habits and lifestyle, but at that point of my life I wasn't exactly thinking logically. Rather than make changes, I rationalized that at least now I knew I just had heartburn and that I hadn't had a heart attack, so let's eat, drink, and be merry. And I did.

Heartburn wasn't the only medical issue that plagued me at night. Countless nights I woke up gasping for air. It wasn't until I was selected for the show that I was diagnosed with sleep apnea. I was so big that the weight on my chest and the fat around my neck was creating enough pressure to literally suffocate me at night and stop my breathing. Since I could count on having at least one episode nearly every night, I found myself fighting to stay awake as long as I could in order to delay the impending agony of my nightly suffocation.

It should come as no surprise that I suffered from severe depression. I was obese, hated my body, couldn't sleep at night, got severe heartburn every time I put something in my mouth, couldn't get a date, felt alone, and could only think of the failures in my life—the list goes on and on. I was not in a good place, although I think I did a pretty good job of covering up my depression with the people who knew me best, even though I was literally falling apart, physically and emotionally. I tried several antidepressant medications, but none of them seemed to help. It wasn't until I had given up taking them, because I was convinced they didn't work, that I found out that alcohol, since it has a depressive effect, basically offset any good the meds could have done for my mental state. My cycle of drinking because I was depressed and being depressed because I drank was a weekly occurrence.

At times my depression was absolutely paralyzing. At home at night, I would rarely turn on lights because I didn't want to see myself. By the age of twenty-nine, I was sleeping at my best friend's house on a regular basis because I didn't want to drive home to an empty house. His couch actually had an indentation where I used to sleep. Looking back, I feel bad for intruding on his life and his wife, who was not only going to school, but also carrying their first daughter at the time.

One of the stranger health problems that I experienced was what I called "phantom pains." My body hurt all over, as if I had bruises everywhere. When I pushed on any part of my body, I would experience a pain that felt like I was pushing on a bruised spot. It was a horrible sensation, and I still don't know the cause to this day. (The pain went away somewhere along the line as my body size and lifestyle improved.) Along with those pains, I also broke out in rashes that were like hives all over my stomach and chest, and I thought it was maybe that I was allergic to certain types of fabrics. In addition, I developed almost purple stretch marks on my belly that were terribly itchy.

These problems were just a few of the ones I encountered prior to being on the show. You would think I would have gone to a doctor to see just how bad things really were, but I didn't, mainly because I was too afraid and embarrassed. To be honest, I didn't want to know at that point in my life; I obviously wasn't ready to make any changes, and deep down I knew that if I were to go see a doctor, he or she would definitely tell me that I needed to change my health habits or I would die.

Fast Forward to the Show, Health-Wise

Fast forward a little bit from the health problems I was just describing. I was cast to be on *The Biggest Loser*, where I got my first physical in nearly ten years. Just as I feared, the doc who examined me said, "If you don't lose weight and change your ways, you will die young." For the first time, though, I was able to see—on paper, in black and white—the actual evidence of the damage that I had been doing to my body beyond the pain and other symptoms that I had been trying so hard to ignore.

My numbers struck fear into me. For starters, I found out that I wasn't just a big guy, but that I was considered "morbidly obese," with a body mass index (BMI) of 48.6. My waist measured fifty five and a quarter inches, which put me at an even higher risk for heart disease. My blood pressure was 155/98, so the doctor immediately put me on meds for that. What's more, I was a pre-diabetic, with elevated fasting insulin and above-normal blood sugar levels. Perhaps the most telling sign of how unhealthy I had become, though, was my abnormal blood fats. My total cholesterol was 230 mg/dl, my triglycerides were 428, my LDL cholesterol was off the charts, and my good HDL cholesterol values were only 41—which wasn't bad, but way too low to compensate for everything else. I also had acid reflux disease and gallbladder colic to round it out. To put it mildly, I was in bad shape, and I wasn't even thirty yet.

That physical exam may have been the most important one of my entire life. Prior to that day, I had only sought out treatment for my depression and had visited the ER once (when I thought I was dying from heartburn). As bleak as things looked, I knew they could only get better, and they did. Probably the most important thing I learned from actually getting a physical was how important it is to know what's going on in your body. By finding out how much damage I was inflicting on my own body, I was able to digest, figuratively, how serious things were with my health. As a man, I had believed that I was too tough to go get a physical. I thought that people who went to the doctor were weak and that the only time you should go to the doctor was for surgery or if you were going to die. Well, I was literally eating and drinking myself to death, and I still wouldn't go see a doctor before the show made me do it.

As I mentioned, my uncle Mark, my dad's brother, died from a heart attack during my time on the Ranch. Although he was only fifty years old, he went to bed one night with what he thought was heartburn and didn't wake up. My uncle left behind his wife, three kids, and several grandkids. He didn't even know it was coming. I don't think anybody really knows when he (or she) is going to have a heart attack, but you can know when you're at risk for one. At the age of twenty-nine, I would have never believed that I might have a heart attack, but I could have easily been just like my uncle, maybe even before reaching the half-century milestone.

If you remember only one thing after you finish this book, I hope it is this: it's important to know your family history when it comes to your health. Whether we like it or not, we inherit a lot from our family, some good and some bad. If we got the genes for bad health, we need to be aware of it and take steps to decrease its possible effects. Listen to your body. If you are feeling unusual pains or have things going on that just don't seem quite right, get them checked out sooner rather than later (or not at all). Lastly, get a physical with a full workup, especially if you are overweight or have a family history of heart disease or diabetes. If you aren't willing to go for yourself, get it done for your family. Of course, we all want to seem invincible for our families and others close to us, but let me tell you, it's really hard to look tough and invincible when you are dead, especially at a young age. Think of

"If you don't lose all the weight, you can't be healthy."

Fiction. Even with small reductions in your weight (such as 5 to 7 percent, or no more than 10 to 15 pounds for most people), which often occur over time as you become more active and make small changes in your dietary patterns, the majority of health benefits can and will be yours. Lifestyle choices play the biggest role in determining whether you develop obesity, pre-diabetes, diabetes, heart disease, high blood pressure, and more. Thankfully, almost all of these conditions can all be improved or prevented altogether without major dieting and significant weight loss. The key things are to start moving your body more, make improvements in your diet, and find ways to effectively manage your stress and depression.

how your family would feel if you didn't wake up tomorrow because of something (even a little thing like sleep apnea caused by being overweight or obese) that could have been prevented with simply a little more knowledge and action on your part.

Know Your Numbers

To find out where you stand in terms of your health, it's important to know some health-related values that you would usually get during an annual checkup. Most of them come from a simple, fasting blood draw (a single vial, usually) at your doctor's office. You should also have your blood pressure measured regularly. If your values are higher than normal, talk to your doctor about what you can do to get them into a better range, and consider making some changes to your lifestyle to improve your health.

	Fasting (Overnight)	Other Times
Blood Glucose (mg/dl)	70-99 (or <120 before all meals)	<180 one hour after meals and <140 two hours after eating
Total Cholesterol (mg/dl)	<200	<180 (even better, especially if you have any other risk factors for heart disease)
HDL-Cholesterol (mg/dl)	>40 for males, >50 for females	>60 (optimal for everyone)
LDL-Cholesterol (mg/dl)	<100	<70 (if at higher risk for heart disease)
Triglycerides (mg/dl)	<150	Varies following meals
Blood Pressure (mm Hg)	<120/<80	Never over 130/85

"Most people with some extra body weight—even the 'pleasantly plump' ones—actually would be considered clinically obese according to body mass index (BMI) guidelines."

Fact. It doesn't take much to be clinically defined as "obese," just a body mass index, or BMI, of 30 or higher. For example, a five-foot-ten-inch male would reach that value at a body weight of just 209 pounds. To be in the normal range, your BMI should be 18.5 to 24.9. "Overweight" is defined as a BMI of 25 to 29.9, and "obese" starts at 30, going up to "morbidly obese" at a value of 40. Muscle mass weighs more than fat at the same volume, so having extra muscle mass will raise your BMI, but don't blame your extra muscle for a BMI that is above the "overweight" range, because muscle doesn't weigh *that* much.

You can easily calculate your BMI yourself. It equals your weight in kilograms divided by the square of your height in meters (wt/ht^2). Take your weight in pounds and divide

➡

by 2.2 to get your weight in kilograms; multiply your height in inches by 0.0254 to get your height in meters. For example, if you weigh 83 kg (182.5 pounds) and are 1.78 meters tall (five foot ten), your BMI is the following: $83/1.78^2 = 83/3.17 = 26.2$. If you'd rather, substitute your pounds and inches in the equation and multiply the answer by 705. Also look for online BMI calculators, such as the one at www.nhlbisupport.com/bmi/bmicalc.htm.

Dr. Sheri's Tips for Staying Motivated to Be Physically Active

- Get yourself an exercise buddy (even a dog that needs to be walked).
- Break your larger goals into smaller, realistic stepping stones (e.g., daily and weekly physical activity goals).
- Use sticker charts or other motivational tools to track your progress, and reward yourself with non-caloric treats or outings for reaching your goals.

- Schedule structured exercise into your day on your calendar or on a "To Do" list, and treat it like a meeting that you just can't miss.

- Plan to do fun physical activities that you really enjoy as often as possible to keep your exercise fun and your motivation high.

- Wear a pedometer (at least occasionally) as a reminder to take more daily steps; try to take at least 10,000 a day, or aim for at least 2,000 a day more than you currently take.

- Have a backup plan that includes alternate activities in case of inclement weather or other barriers to your planned exercise.

- Distract yourself while you exercise by reading a book or magazine, watching TV, listening to music or a book on tape, or talking with a friend or on the phone.

- Don't start out exercising too intensely or you're likely to get discouraged or injured and quit.

- If you get out of your normal routine and have trouble getting restarted, simply take small steps in that direction until you're back on track.

CHAPTER 8

Keep the Weight Off—Forever

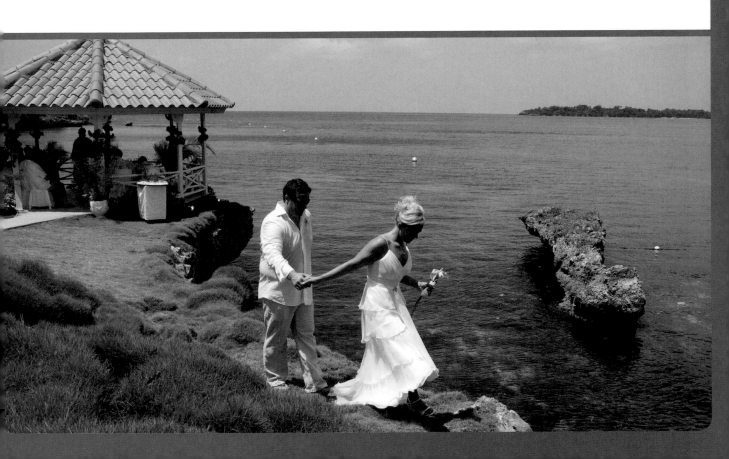

What *The Biggest Loser* show usually fails to relay to people is that losing weight is only half the battle, often the easier half. If you think you're alone in regaining some of the weight that you worked so hard to lose, think again. In reality, most people gain the weight back after they lose it, and then go on another diet, and regain it—you get the idea. We've all seen Oprah and other celebrities do it. It's so common that it has its own name, "yo-yo dieting," because your weight is constantly going up and down.

There was a special *Biggest Loser* reunion show on not long ago, and they did bring a select few of the past winners and participants back on to ask them each the question, "Did you keep the weight off?" Of course, I happen to know for a fact that they only considered asking a limited number of contestants to return because the rest had regained too much weight after losing it during their respective seasons. Why is gaining the weight back so commonplace,

and what can you do about it? Hopefully, this final chapter will give you some tips that you can take to the weight loss bank for the rest of your life.

My Life After *The Biggest Loser 2*

Today my life is dramatically different than it was before or during the show. It's not just myself that I have to worry about anymore, and I don't have the luxury of being selfish because of the other commitments in my life. I have a wife whom I adore and a son who has changed my life forever, for the better. When I can't find the motivation to stay healthy for myself alone, I just think about what I need to do to make sure I'm around for a long time to enjoy seeing my son grow up and to have the opportunity to grow old with my wife.

When I had all the time to work out a ridiculous amount every day, I never gave much thought to what it would be

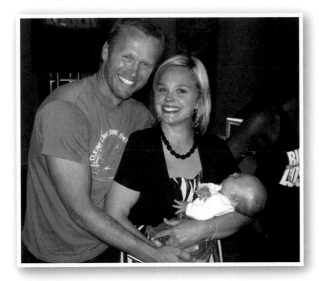

Suzy with our friend and trainer, Bob Harper, and our son, Rex.

like when I didn't have that kind of time anymore. The year following the show was hectic, to say the least. I traveled around the country making appearances at various engagements. Only a few months after Suzy and I started dating, I proposed to her, I moved to the West Coast, and we got married. Because my livelihood depended upon me being in good shape, it was easy to fit in my workouts. I learned quickly the importance of planning ahead. Also, I got to know many of the busiest airports, including the places where I could find something halfway healthy to eat. I knew that I had to keep on making good choices while I was on the road. For instance, when I arrived at the hotel I was staying at, I went for a run; after sitting in a seat all day on a long flight, the last thing I really wanted to do was work out, but I always felt better afterward. (A little side note, I found out the hard way that it is a good idea to know where you are running. I got lost on a run one time, so every time after that, I just ran straight out from the hotel and ran straight back in order to avoid getting hopelessly lost.)

The other pitfall I had to avoid was ordering the wrong things at restaurants. Many times, the people that set up the event took me out to dinner, usually to the best place in town. Each restaurant had its own dish that people told me I just had to try. I usually politely explained that I need to stick to my diet plan. There were times

"Most people keep the weight off."

Fiction. The reality of dieting is that over the long haul, it just does *not* work for most people. Not only does it become progressively harder to lose weight the longer you diet (thus making it harder for you to stay motivated), but also at least 90 percent of dieters who have successfully lost weight ultimately regain the pounds that they struggled to shed. In reality, most people gain back even more weight than they originally lost, regardless of which diet they followed.

Even if you do keep your weight under control, it's common to regain some of what you lost while dieting. Even among successful weight-loss maintainers in the National Weight Control Registry (see box later in this chapter), some weight gain was common during the two years after they joined the registry, and recovery from even minor weight regain was uncommon. Those who regained less in the first year, though, fared better, as did those who reported fewer and less severe bouts of depression, which gives you another good reason to work on your emotional as well as physical health.

when the specialty of the house fit with my diet, but other times I had to respectfully decline. Learning how to say "no" is an excellent skill to master. No one ever appeared to be offended when I said that I need to eat a certain way or that I chose not to do something because it didn't fit into my lifestyle. I maintained my weight pretty easily the whole time I was on the road by simply developing a plan and sticking to it.

Suzy and I got married in September 2006. That beautiful sunny day in Jamaica surrounded by our family, we made a commitment to love and cherish each other. We also committed to be healthy together. Even on our honeymoon we got our workouts in. It was more crucial to be active there because our resort, the Grand Lido, was an amazing all-inclusive resort where the food was not only plentiful, but also amazingly prepared. I thoroughly enjoyed every meal, but got away with it only because we stayed active.

Let's Be Real: Even I Gained Some Back

Let me tell you more about my story since *The Biggest Loser 2*, in case you forgot that I'm just a normal guy. I have been a motivational and keynote speaker since 2005, when the show brought me so much publicity for my weight loss success. To this day, I book my own speaking engagements. I don't get paid unless I have some, so my income depends on continuing to be motivational to others. As you would expect, I am usually invited to speak because I lost weight and people want to learn how they can, too.

I would love to think that people ask me to speak to them because I am a nice guy with a great personality. The truth is that they want me as their speaker for the way I look—not because I have movie star looks, but because I was able to go from being morbidly obese to an average size. My career and my family's livelihood depend upon my staying in shape and living the lifestyle I teach to others. Why would anyone who lost weight want to make a career out of speaking about it? Statistics overwhelmingly show that nearly everyone who loses weight gains it back. Well, let me tell you, there have been some times I have questioned myself and my new career, when I found myself thinking and starting to act like the old me, the Matt who would rather sit around than work out, the one who was

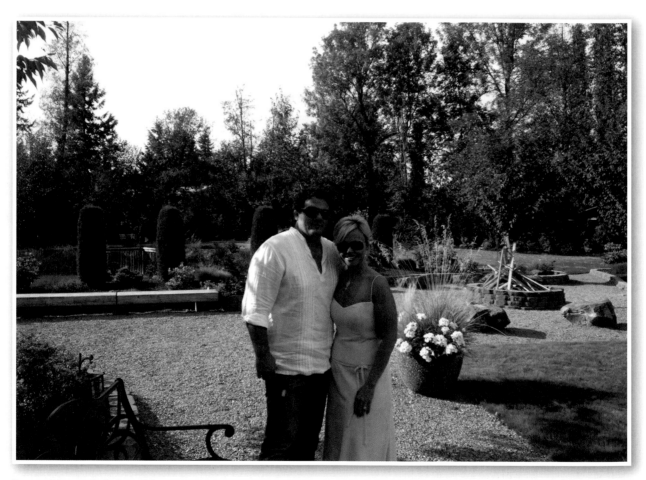

Suzy and I at a relative's wedding

lazy enough to let work come to him rather than seeking it out.

People's businesses fail because they start taking it easy and get complacent. I guess I'm no different than most people in that respect. My first year as a full-time speaker was extremely busy. When my wife gave birth to our son in the summer of 2007, I decided to take some time off. With a new baby, I found it easier to skip workouts, and I soon found myself packing on some of the pounds that I had worked so hard to take off. I justified it by saying that it was just part of the process that all new dads go through. I mean, after all, I was getting awakened so often during the night by the baby crying that it just wasn't realistic for me to expect myself to stick with my usual workouts. A person would have to be superhuman to pull that off, right? My mistake! In retrospect, I finally acknowledged that people continue to run multimillion-dollar companies after having newborns, and many others continue to go to the gym even when losing lots of sleep from nighttime feedings. In fact, it's not uncommon for people to be able to adapt and continue doing the things they need to in order to stay on top of their game.

I did an interview with Larry King on his show shortly after my son was born. It wasn't until I saw myself on national TV again that I realized I was definitely heading for trouble. I talked about how I wanted to be a role model for my son, how we wanted to be a healthy family, and how I was working on various projects. More important than what I said, though, was what I saw on the TV. In watching it later, I saw myself as others saw me—not those close to me, but people who had never seen me before or who may not have known my story—and I didn't think that they would be impressed by my size, even though I was nowhere near as big as I had been when I started the show.

My first thought after seeing myself was, "What am I doing?" I had spent the last two years traveling around the country and making great money by sharing my story. I love my job, and I really believe that my calling is to speak and help others by relating my own experiences. But for the first time in years, I saw a brief glimpse of the old sales rep Matt, the guy who could talk and sound professional, but whose appearance said otherwise. "Terrified" may very well be the best description of how I felt that night after seeing myself. I felt the terror of potentially letting my career slip through my hands, of not being able to provide for my family, and, most of all, of reverting to my old ways. In my mind, I had begun to commit what in the financial world would equate to filing for bankruptcy. I knew that if I didn't get it back together immediately, I would have to find a new line of work. The old Matt would have said, "Well, you blew it again. I knew it was just a matter of time." But the new Matt was saying in a louder voice, "Boy, you better get it together and quick! How can you turn this lesson into something good?"

Nearly every day you hear stories about how a person takes over a failing business and turns it around. After reworking systems, changing policy, and perhaps doing some house cleaning, the company takes back off and prospers. I realized that I needed to do some house cleaning, and the cleaning began with my own body. I knew that if I weren't physically fit, my credibility, my marketability, and my career were essentially nonexistent. I needed to get serious. Right after that, I didn't take any engagements and I stopped doing interviews. I got into the gym and treated my workouts like they were my job, essentially telling myself that I was investing in my company. I set a target date to reach my goal body weight, and then I booked a speaking engagement for right after that date. I knew I wouldn't be able to do any events unless I was looking and feeling fit. Giving myself a concrete date and a contract that was dependent upon my reaching my goal made me work as hard as I ever have.

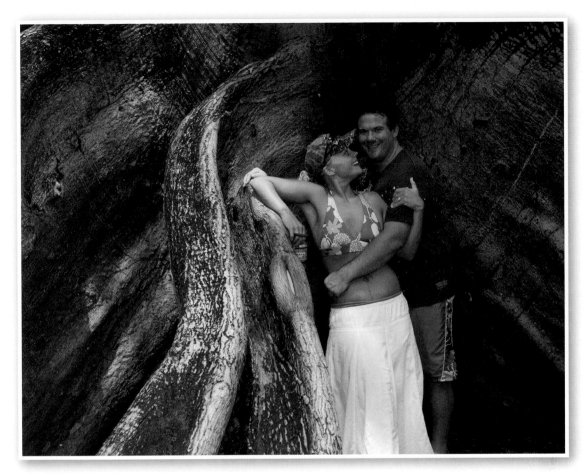

Posing by a huge tree at the Grand Lido in Negril, Jamaica

I am a real person, and I intend to continue using my experiences to help others take control of their health. I get e-mails nearly every day from people asking me how they can change their lives like I have changed mine. In essence, it comes down to constantly learning and evolving. Although I created my own setbacks by gaining some weight back, the difference is that I got serious and corrected it before it went too far.

The Dangers of Yo-Yo Dieting (or Constantly Losing and Regaining the Weight)

One main problem with large amounts of weight loss is that, if they're not careful, typical dieters lose about 75 percent fat and 25 percent muscle. Losing the fat is good, but losing your muscle mass is not, because if you ever gain the weight back (which as many as 90 percent of dieters do), your weight regain may be up to 85 percent fat and only 15 percent muscle, making you actually more fat (percentage-wise) than before you dieted. Each time you lose muscle and gain fat back in its place, your metabolism slows down, making it that much easier to gain more weight even if your caloric intake stays the same. What's more, if you yo-yo diet over your lifetime (frequently cycling between weight loss and regain) and lose muscle each time, when you're older, you may not have enough muscle left to carry your extra body weight around, thereby reducing how well you feel and can function.

Rather than just throwing in the towel, I stood up and fought for my successes. I have also learned that I will have to fight this battle for the rest of my life. As became apparent that night on *Larry King Live*, no matter how hard I have worked in the past or what results I achieved, resting on my laurels will only get me right back to where

I started: a bad place that I don't want to return to, ever.

How Did I Turn It Around?

When my wife became pregnant and I took some time off, I attributed the weight gain to the old standby of sympathetic pregnancy gain, but truth be known, I just let myself be lazy for a while. I figured no one was going to see me, so what difference did it make if I gained a few extra pounds? Well, shortly after the birth of our son, when people saw the weight I had gained during that appearance on *Larry King Live,* I was embarrassed. I had to make sure that my career didn't end the night of that interview. The first thing I did was to evaluate what was happening to me. The interview was over and my physical appearance that night could not be changed, but what could change was me. I had to get to work immediately. I couldn't dwell on what had gone wrong, but instead needed to think about what I still had: a book deal, people wanting me to speak to

motivate others, and, most importantly, my family.

At that point, it was time to implement my own ideas and the lessons that I had been sharing with others over the last two years. Rather than lie down and hide and quit like I had so many times throughout the years, I decided to accept responsibility and to fight. I took a long look at myself and then came to some conclusions.

First, I looked like I looked. Millions of people saw me that night and were going to have their opinions. I could not change that—it was a done deal. I now had to implement the things I had learned on the *Biggest Loser* show and get myself back to a place where I felt good physically. That would be easy enough, and I was motivated to do it.

Second, I needed to understand why I was letting my weight increase even though I knew it could mean the end of my new-found career. The only thing I could think of was self-pity, the same thing that had gotten me on the show in the first place—I used to be something and now look at me, poor me. I had rationalized that I was a husband and a dad now, so why did I need to keep my weight down? I got selfish and threw a little pity party. I thought about how mean people were with their comments on the Internet and vowed, "I'll show them." I showed them all right—that they were right when they predicted that I was going to fall back into old habits and go back to where I started.

Those negative thoughts could have consumed me, but I chose not to let them take over my life again. This was my new life, and I was not going to go back to my old ways. Fortunately, I was able to implement the very lessons that I had conveyed to hundreds of thousands of people as a speaker. *I recognized my old thought patterns and implemented new ones!* That's right. All of the negative thoughts I listed above did go through my head, but I was able to quickly replace them with more positive

ones that were conducive to getting back on track. It helped me to recognize this as yet another opportunity to learn as well as teach.

I have seen studies that say nearly 90 percent of people who lose weight regain all or most of their weight back within a couple of years. I had kept off nearly one hundred pounds for over two years, so I was ahead of the curve in that respect, but I needed to get myself back to where I felt comfortable. How was I going to do that? By using the techniques that helped me lose the weight in the first place, I reasoned. I couldn't diet and exercise just when I felt like it. They had to be a priority. I couldn't be complacent and say, "At least I've kept off some weight." That type of thinking is an invitation to gain weight, and that is just what I had done.

The next thing I did was to ask myself, "How can I help others through this experience?" Just because I had lost weight in front of a national TV audience didn't make my weight issues any less difficult. I still struggle as much as anyone else with temptation, and I fight the desire to skip workouts. Weight issues don't just disappear when you lose some body fat. I decided the best way that I could help others was by breaking the cycle of weight gain and loss

myself. I want to teach people that breaking this cycle begins from within, and I knew that I couldn't help others if I didn't first help myself.

By accepting weight gain as a normal part of the process, I imposed a prison sentence on myself. I would serve my time

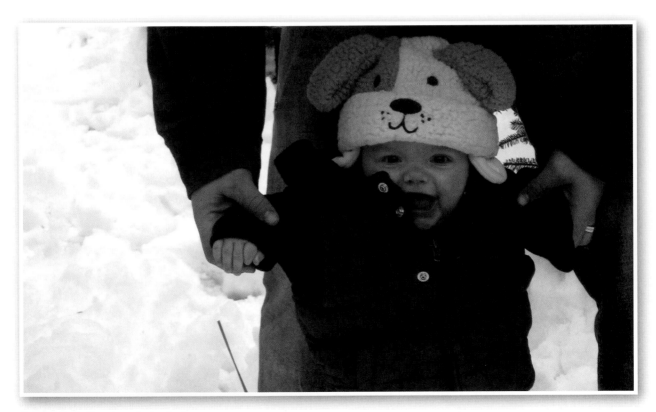

Our son Rex's first time playing in the snow.

by constantly gaining weight or losing weight, making it a lifelong sentence. Not only that, but if I didn't break the cycle, I would be imposing the same upon my family as well. My wife would have to serve time with me, and one day, my son and his family would have it imposed upon them as well. I did not want to be responsible for my family's lifetime struggle with weight. I decided that the cycle of weight gain and weight loss was going to end here, with me—not because I was tired of hearing about how fat I had gotten from perfect strangers who were hiding behind their computer screens, but rather because I love my family and would not wish my struggles on them.

I acted upon this decision by refusing to feel sorry for myself. Understanding that healthy eating and daily exercise were simply going to be a part of my life, I made them as routine as breathing. You have to breathe to live; for me to live the way I want, exercise and a healthy diet are as vital as breathing.

How often do you think about breathing? Rarely, if ever, would be my guess. Now I have gotten to the point where I go to the gym and make healthy choices without giving it much thought. When something becomes so routine that you rarely think of it, you have formed a habit. Healthy habits are good because they make once difficult chores like exercising much more enjoyable. Not only do such habits help me, living in this manner will make it easier for my young son to adopt my good habits rather than my bad ones. The cool thing about healthy, good habits is that over time they will naturally override the bad.

Today I maintain a healthy weight along with my active and beautiful wife and son. Physical activity and a healthy diet are two very important aspects of our family. I can say that the best lesson I learned from putting some weight back on is that I don't have to keep it on. By making good choices and forming healthy, lifelong habits, I can maintain a healthy weight and enjoy my life. Had I not gained back the weight when I did, I might not have recognized that I still had some work to do. By taking care of it early, I was able to overcome one more hurdle. Because of my experiences, I have no worries about my son's life and am confident that he will not have to endure the body weight struggles that both his dad and his mother did.

I think my greatest gift as a speaker is my ability to relate to others and to honestly share my personal stories. Because I made mistakes and then corrected them, I am able to do my job even better.

Losing the Weight for Good: More Lessons from the NWCR

Over the past decade, the National Weight Control Registry (NWCR) has tracked individuals who have lost at least 30 pounds *and* kept the weight off for at least a year. Keeping lost weight off for a year is actually quite uncommon, even among successful dieters, since you're most likely to regain the weight you lost within the first six months after the diet ends. The NWCR members have lost between thirty and three hundred pounds and have managed their weight loss for between one and sixty-six years, so there's a lot of diversity among them. Some lost their weight rapidly, while others have done so slowly over a number of years.

➡

Their results confirm what exercise professionals like Dr. Sheri have known all along: physical activity matters. It doesn't appear to make any difference what method or weight loss plan the successful dieters used to lose weight. What matters most are the three lifestyle habits that almost all of them adopt to maintain their lower body weight. First, they continue to be conscientious about what they eat (focusing on more healthful, lower-calorie foods in appropriate portions, with limited consumption of fast foods, and a moderate fat intake), and most weigh themselves at least once a week. Second, they start their day off right with a balanced and healthy breakfast (high-fiber cereals and fruit top the list). Third, and likely most important, 90 percent of them *exercise almost daily*, on average for about an hour, and expend about 2,000 calories a week being physically active. Even in studies on diabetes prevention, people who participate by making lifestyle changes are only successful at keeping any lost weight off (and preventing the onset of diabetes) if they continue to exercise regularly and monitor the amount of calories (particularly fat) that they eat. So, if you want to maintain your weight loss, get up off the couch and go for a walk (and do it again tomorrow, and the next day, and the next)—but eat your breakfast first.

Lessons I Have Learned of Late

If my new career had ended that night of my interview with Larry King, I still would have had my family, and that makes me a lucky man. The rest of it is anything but luck. Let me share with you some of the lessons I have learned of late.

Lesson 1: Know your priorities

My priority is my family, and in order to take care of them, I have to take care of myself first. In essence, I have to be my number one priority—not in a selfish way, but in a way that allows me to be productive and successful. I don't believe it is possible to truly take care of others unless you are first able to take care of yourself.

Lesson 2: Focus on what you have, not on what you think you don't

It is easy to think of what you supposedly lost because of an incident during your career. The night after my Larry King interview, my first thought was that I had lost everything and that my career was over. It wasn't. Only in my mind had I lost anything. Think about it: I will never actually know if I lost any speaking engagements because of the way I looked that night on television. Not one person called me up and said, "Mr. Hoover, I just wanted to say that I saw you on TV and because you looked a little heavy, we aren't going to have you do an event for us." You can't lose something you never had. Growing up in Iowa, I remember farmers talking about how they had lost money because of the market conditions. "If I had sold last week, I would have made out pretty good, but I lost it since I didn't," one would say. Do you see the mindset I'm talking about? The farmer still had his corn or cows, so he hadn't actually lost a thing, yet he let the idea of what he could have had instead negatively impact his mindset.

What did I have? I still had a book deal. Although my coauthor, publisher, and literary agent asked me what was up with my weight, they were willing to let me go through with the project. I needed to come through because a lot of people were counting on me to not only get back on track, but also to stay on track once I got there. So that was one thing that I still had and could use to motivate myself. Another thing I still had was my story, and through it, a career. My job is to tell my story—and to tell it truthfully. This minor setback just turned out to be another aspect of what I had to share. I thought about how I would be able to relate my experiences in a way that would allow others to benefit from them as well. It was a no-brainer, as they say. People

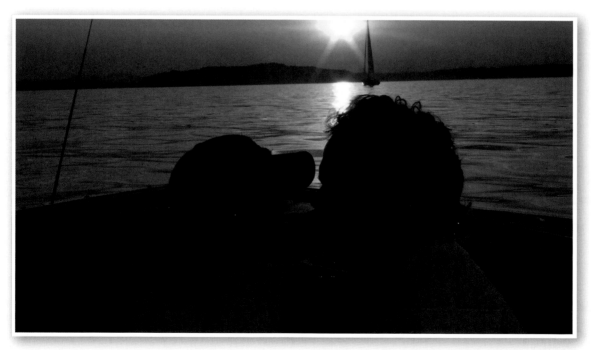

Enjoying the Puget Sound sunset on our boat

lose weight and the majority of them gain it back (and then some). I wanted to use my own experience to illustrate how we need to keep fighting, especially after experiencing the short-lived joy of achieving an initial goal. I needed to model the importance of continuing to do the same things that created the initial positive results in order to sustain them. In short, I decided to use my own experiences as evidence for this principle.

Lesson 3: Be honest with yourself

It would have been easy for me to convince myself that things weren't that bad—heck, I had done it for years when I was severely overweight, so I had lots of practice. Besides, this time I had kept nearly one hundred pounds off for almost two years. Most people would be thrilled with that, but I wasn't. I knew deep down that if I didn't react immediately, my weight would eventually climb back to where I started. Even though I had gained back more weight than I would have liked, people told me on a regular basis how good I looked. Strangers approached my wife and I recently, apparently fans of ours, to tell us how great we still looked and how we inspired them to lose weight themselves. While I'm glad that they had decided to take care of themselves, deep down I was thinking, "If you only knew how fat I am right now." I couldn't let myself become complacent in the face of compliments.

Many times, unfortunately, we let ourselves believe that we are better off simply because things aren't as bad as they use to be. This may be the case, but imagine how good things could become if we were to honestly evaluate ourselves on a regular basis. When it comes down to it, we're the only ones who really know how well we are performing. I got pretty good reviews when I was in sales, but I knew I could have done better if I had expended a little more effort. Are you putting a good effort forward in whatever your endeavor is at this moment? If you are, then you're doing great, and I applaud you. If you aren't, imagine how different things could be if you would be honest with yourself and commit to refocusing in the direction you'd really like to be going instead.

Lesson 4: Get over it

It is much easier to dwell on what went wrong than it is to take the steps to fix it—or is it? Actually, I believe that it takes just as much energy to be miserable as it does to feel good. I can remember thinking about all of the things that had gone wrong in my life and trying to figure out whose fault it was. I didn't become a national champion in college; today I can think, If I only had done this and this, things would have been different. The reality of it is that I can never go back and be a national champ for the Iowa Hawkeyes. I didn't achieve that goal and now there is nothing I can do about it.

You might be thinking, "Well, that's a no-brainer, Matt. Why are you still talking about college?" I know I can't go back, although it took me a long time to accept that fact. Now ask yourself, What am I still holding on to? Do you cling to failures or unachieved goals? Until I was able to finally let go of my past and the things I didn't accomplish, I wasn't able to move forward. It's hard to see what's coming if you are always looking back. I felt pain and I blamed others for it, but I had to get over it. One of the best things I have ever done for myself was coming to terms with my past and what I could and could not do about it. If you can't change it now, learn from it, let it go, and move on.

Lesson 5: Take responsibility

Many of us choose to blame others, perhaps because it makes us feel better about our current situation. Not taking responsibility for our own actions allows us to hold on to past pain or anger, as well as giving us a built-in excuse for making the same mistakes in the future. When I left school only a few credits short of a degree, I blamed the professors for not giving me enough attention. When

I quit the Iowa wrestling team, I blamed my injuries. When I drank, I blamed my problems. The reason I had the problems in the first place was never my fault.

In actuality, the majority of my problems were my fault—mine and mine only. I was the one who didn't go to class and, therefore, had to drop out when I failed; I stayed out all night partying and drinking and then went to wrestling practice tired and got hurt— though I never came home after a night of drinking with a sore shoulder from people twisting my arm to drink. The choices were mine, and I was the one who had to deal with the consequences. Until I was willing to take responsibility, I found myself making similar mistakes over and over again. When I finally realized that I had made every decision, be it good or bad, I began to understand the importance of taking responsibility for myself and my actions.

No one but us has the ability to determine how we respond to a situation. We ultimately dictate which direction our path in life will go. We can blame others and stay right where we are, or we can accept what we have done, take responsibility, and move forward. Taking responsibility is the next step in moving past your past.

Lesson 6: Make a plan

Here's an example from my own life about the importance of planning ahead in reaching goals. One day my wife and I decided we were going to take a road trip to see the ocean. I had been living in Washington state for several months and had yet to see the Pacific Coast. I love water and had seen the ocean in California, but I wanted to see how the landscape and the water were different in my new home state. That night, after Suzy was done working, we hopped in the car and headed west. We didn't take a map; we just headed out. I had asked a few people how long it took to get to the ocean, and all of them said it took two and a half to three hours. We drove and talked, and after a while we realized we hadn't seen a single sign indicating where to turn. I asked Suzy if anything looked familiar, but she didn't think so. The next sign said we were getting very close to Oregon. I knew at this point we were not going to get to the ocean or an oceanfront hotel anytime soon.

Then I decided to turn on the navigation system in our car. The GPS said I needed to turn around and go back several miles in the opposite direction. Well, being a man on a mission, I decided that if I kept going just a little farther, the system would realize that it was wrong and that there was a quicker way. There wasn't. My wife fell asleep while I drove, and we ended up in Portland, Oregon. You don't have to be a geographer to look at a map and see that Portland is nearly straight south of Seattle and that the Pacific Ocean is directly west. I had gone the wrong direction for over two hours. Fortunately, when I got to Portland, the GPS did reset, just as I had planned some time ago. I followed directions and headed toward the coast. We stopped at a hotel at around one o'clock in the morning, still over an hour from the ocean.

The next morning we headed out. Instead of following the GPS, I once again decided to make my own way back up to Washington to reach the destination I had originally decided on. We drove for hours, but unfortunately we never did make it to see the Washington coast. You may be asking, "Why would someone start out on a trip to a place that he has never been without first looking at a map and coming up with a plan to get there?" A better question is, "Why wouldn't someone who has a satellite-guided GPS system, which is extremely accurate, actually use it?" It's because most of us (at least us guys), want to prove that we know what is best for us, even if we know we are lost. I was going in the wrong direction, but I didn't want to admit it.

In situations much more serious than a drive to the ocean, we often allow ourselves to continue in the wrong direction when all the clues tell us to turn around. My trip was pretty much doomed from the moment I decided I didn't need a map or a plan to find the Pacific Ocean. The ironic thing is that although nearly everyone knows he or she needs to develop a plan before beginning a journey, often people will fail to do that simple thing. Think of the last time you started on a journey without a solid plan. How did that work for you? Did you achieve your goal? The most successful people I know are meticulous planners. They know what they need to do and when it needs to be done in order to achieve their goals. The lesson in this case is that the only way to reach your destination is to plan for it, not just leave it to chance or your own misguided notions.

Lesson 7: Don't be afraid of change

I was extremely afraid of changing anything about myself, even during the roughest patches in my life. On some level, I must have known that if I made a few changes in my behavior, things could turn around for me. Even so, I chose to stay where I was. My problem was that the longer I chose not to change, the further into despair I fell. The deeper and deeper fell, the less I wanted to attempt making any changes for the better.

I don't buy into the idea that a person can stay the same. Life doesn't, and neither can you. If you are not trying to move forward, whether in business, sports, or a relationship, you will eventually begin to slip backward. Change is a good thing. When I got serious about losing weight, I had to change my environment. I had to go to a place where I could focus on myself and the task at hand. After the show, I changed careers, even though I wasn't sure how it was going to go. But I knew that I needed some aspects of my life to be completely different. It was a great move, and I'm glad I did it. If I hadn't, I would not have met and married my wife and, in turn, had my little boy. Change is *good*—and if

"Where you lose the weight from matters."

Fact. Visceral fat, which is the fat deep within your abdomen that makes up most of a "beer belly," has more negative impact on your health and your metabolism than the subcutaneous (below your skin) variety. If you have a choice of losing one or the other, you definitely want to get rid of the intra-abdominal type. Here is where exercise clearly prevails. Dieting alone, although it reduces subcutaneous and total belly fat, does not appear to eliminate much visceral fat or the extra fat stored in muscle. Only if you exercise regularly—regardless of whether you actually lose any body weight—will you lose unhealthy visceral fat. If you exercise without dieting, you'll retain your muscle mass, and if you exercise and diet, you'll lose less muscle than with dieting alone. So, if you have to choose between exercise and dieting for improving your health, choose exercise.

you want the life that you desire, it's necessary. The time to start is now.

Biggest Real World Challenges According to Matt and Suzy

With the amount of weight that Suzy and I have lost between us, we have learned a thing or two about what it takes to keep it off and what is most likely to trip us up. I'd like to share some of our joint challenges, and then Suzy has a few of her own to add.

Joint challenge 1: Food is necessary to live

Alcoholics don't have to drink in order to stay alive. They don't have to go into a bar unless they choose to. They can avoid the places where they're most likely to give in to their addictions. But you have to eat to stay alive, and if you have an addiction to food, a simple task like going into the grocery store can be difficult. What can you do? To avoid a major meltdown, go shopping with a plan, and stick to it. Don't go to the store when you're hungry—you're more likely to buy empty calories that sabotage your goals. Have a list and follow it; a list can minimize the time you spend in the store and reduce the chance you'll choose things you don't need. Back to the alcoholic example—you wouldn't send an alcoholic into a liquor store and tell him to just hang out. The same goes for the grocery store. Don't stand around and stare at all the things you know are not good for you.

If it is simply too difficult to contain yourself in a store, consider buying online. Many stores now offer to deliver the items that you order without leaving your home, and using this service is definitely worth looking into. The cost of the service will probably be less than you might spend on

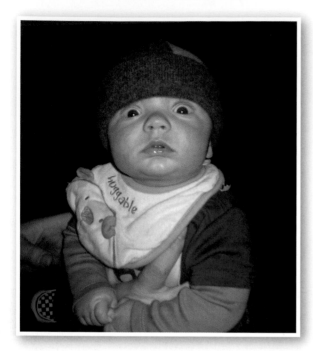

Our little Rex. What are you staring at?

even business. "Let's have a power lunch," or "Let's get some coffee," are common phrases, and we think nothing of it when asked to meet someone at a restaurant. Suzy and I eat out at least once a week, but that doesn't mean that all bets are off when it comes to our food choices. If you start paying attention, you'll find that all restaurants offer at least one healthy choice, and many are more than willing to accommodate a special request that will make an item healthier. For example, ask for your salad dressing on the side, or ask to hold the butter, sour cream, or other calorie-laden condiment. You are paying for a service and should expect to receive service to your liking.

Another strategy is to tell others what your goals are; they can help keep you accountable for your food choices. Many people get frustrated and may feel like others don't care about their goals, when in fact they haven't shared them with their friends, family, and colleagues. Don't expect help if you don't ask for it!

impulse items that end up in the cart in a weak moment—or two.

Joint challenge 2: Going out to eat

Many people think that once you begin a diet plan, enjoying a night out on the town is out of the question. In our society, restaurants serve many purposes: social, celebratory, and

Another option if you aren't ready to eat out is to invite people over to your house. Then you can control your environment and what goes on the dinner plates. It's one of our favorite strategies. We love having people over to grill. No one has ever said to us, "I can't believe you guys are feeding us healthy food," even though that's what we do, and no one turns us down when invited back to our house again. If you go somewhere else to eat, such as a party at someone else's house, you can also bring your own food for a side. Not only will you know that there will be something there for you to eat, but it's a nice gesture to bring something when visiting someone else's home.

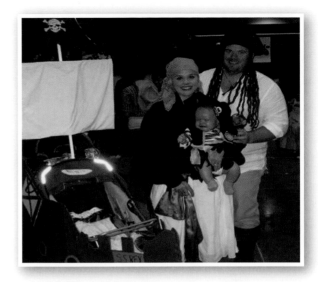

ARGGH! Rex's first Halloween.

on is using moderation. Decide ahead of time that you will only have a certain amount of food, and then stay away from the area where the food is to avoid being tempted.

Joint challenge 3: Holidays

Holidays are tough enough for everyone, but they're especially hard for those of us who struggle with our weight. Once again, planning is essential to stay on track. One thing you should always plan

A difficult holiday that many people overlook is Halloween. The candy hits the shelves in September and what do we do? We "plan ahead" by picking up a bag whenever we are at the store so we can be sure that all of the little trick-or-treaters will

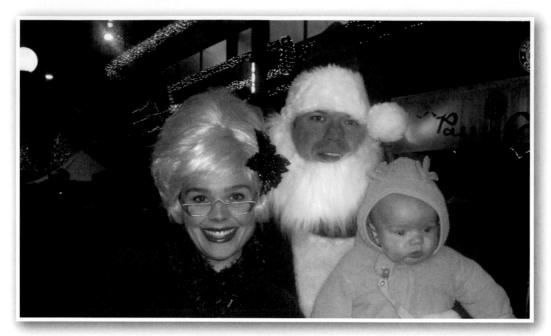

Rex's first 5K. We dressed up as the Clauses for the annual Seattle Jingle Bell Run.

have an abundance of selections. The kids just have to have candy, don't they? What will they ever do without it? We don't want them to have to go without candy on Halloween! Why not just tell them that there is no Santa Claus?

Halloween arrives, and we get prepared for the big night. Pumpkins, check; scary mask, check; candy ... candy, where is all that candy we have been buying? It's nowhere to be found because we ate it all. A piece here, a piece there. We take some to work, it slowly disappears, and we fill the container up again. By the time the holiday actually arrives, we have consumed countless bags of candy. Well, nowadays when the kids stop at our house, they get either a mini container of play dough or a pencil.

We don't wake up the next morning with hundreds of pencils or containers of play dough all over the yard from kids throwing our treats away like you see at the houses that give out crappy candy. The moral of this story is that when you do the things that you feel are right, most people will respect your actions (even kids).

Suzy's challenge 1: What do I do if my husband won't work out with me or doesn't like to work out at the same time I do?

Work out anyway. You can't make someone do something he doesn't want to. I like to work out early in the morning; Matt doesn't. This actually works for us, because Matt can watch our baby (that means the early morning feeding, too) while I get my time in at the gym and then have my morning Starbucks coffee. I have the chance for some alone time and to get ready for what's to come. It's a great way to start the day. In other words, don't use your husband or significant other as a reason to hold yourself back from getting the exercise that is so important to keeping your weight under control.

Suzy's challenge 2: My husband doesn't need to diet and I do all the cooking. How can I get him on board?

If you prepare the meals, prepare them your way and let him decide if he wants to eat or not. That sounds a little harsh, but that's the way it goes sometimes. If he is set in his ways, slowly begin making substitutions and let him get used to them. When you can get the family to start eating healthier, you reduce some of your own struggles. Again, asking for help may be the best approach to this challenge. If you have the chance, like we do with Rex, start out with only healthy foods in your diet, and then your kids will grow up not expecting anything different.

Suzy's challenge 3: You're pregnant!

First, congratulations! Second, you are *not* eating for two! Our midwife was quick to dispel that myth and told us that I only needed about three hundred extra calories a day during my pregnancy. I'm sure opinions vary from doctor to doctor, but our son turned out just fine. I literally worked out until the week Rex was born. In most cases, working out and keeping your body in good shape will only help your pregnancy. Our son was born three weeks early and was perfectly healthy. I am only speaking from my own experience, so consult your physician before exercising while pregnant.

I know it's a personal choice, but you might want to know that one of the best ways to take off any extra baby weight after pregnancy is to breastfeed your baby. It takes about five hundred calories a day to feed your baby, which increases how many calories your body uses up and helps the extra

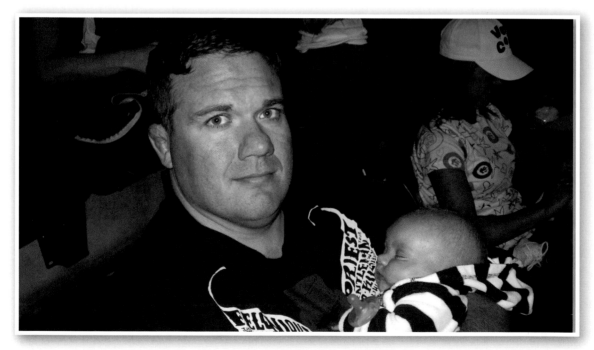

Rex's first trip to the Barnum and Bailey Circus. He could hardly contain his excitement.

"Starting your kids dieting early helps keep them thin throughout their lives."

Fiction. Studies show that putting your kids on strict diets promotes weight gain instead of keeping them thinner. For teens in particular, dieting to control weight is not only ineffective, but may actually promote weight gain. It appears that binge-eating is more common in both girls and boys who diet, and teenage dieters gain more weight than non-dieters in the longer term. How is this possible? One reason is that dieting may improve metabolic efficiency, which means that your body requires fewer calories. Cutting back dramatically on calorie intake is also usually followed by a period of over-eating and bingeing, which leads to weight gain. If your teens aren't severely overweight, it's better to focus instead on getting them more physically active and staying that way.

fat (that almost everyone has) melt right off. The trick to breastfeeding well is to make sure that you stay hydrated by drinking plenty of water and eating enough protein and calcium to keep your milk supply up and full of the nutrients your baby needs. Breast milk is the best food for your newborn—almost exclusively for the first six months of

Is It Safe to Lose Weight When You're Over Sixty?

How old you are when you lose weight isn't something that most people think about, but according to aging specialist Dr. John E. Morley, it's probably not safe to lose large amounts of body weight when you're older than sixty. One main problem with significant weight loss after you reach middle-age or older is that you invariably lose some muscle along with the fat. If you gain weight afterward, a larger percentage of weight is regained as body fat. Losing muscle also lowers your metabolism—an occurrence that we all have to fight against as we age—making it easier to gain weight even if you eat the same number of calories after your diet. When you lose excessive amounts of body weight when you're older, you can also more easily develop protein energy malnutrition, which is caused by taking in less protein (and calories) than your body needs. It can lead to all sorts of physical problems (e.g., pressure ulcers, anemia, hip fractures, infections, and muscle weakness) that can make your health suffer.

Another reason to avoid weight loss in later life is that losing weight causes stored fats to be released into your bloodstream, where they can contribute to the bad type of cholesterol, potentially contributing to heart disease, plaque formation, and blood clots. You're also releasing whatever has been stored in your fat tissue along with it, including a lifetime of accumulated toxins like PCBs and DDEs from insecticides, which can actually lead to nerve damage. Similarly, many medications are stored in fat tissue, and weight loss releases more of them as well, which can make the doses that you're exposed to excessively high and potentially harmful to your health.

his or her life—and breastfed babies are less likely to become overweight or obese children or adults, which means that you can help start your child off on the right path to maintaining a normal body weight.

Matt's Answers to Some of the Questions He's Been Asked

I have spoken all over the country and have had the opportunity to meet some great people. At the end of every engagement, I open up my talk for questions. Some questions have been really good, and I would like share a few of them with you.

Question 1: I have tried everything to lose weight. Do you have any suggestions?

Try one more time. Start with realistic and attainable goals. If you have a hundred pounds to lose, start with the goal of losing five. By setting a small goal first, you will be less likely to become frustrated and give up. The task of losing a large amount of weight can seem insurmountable at times. Take it slow and steady. I lost 157 pounds over the course of nine months, and I personally feel that it was way too fast. Many of the people that I have met who had lasting results took their time, and they made their weight loss more permanent that way.

Question 2: I can't afford to join a gym and buy expensive healthy food. How can I get healthy if I can't afford it?

This is one of my favorite questions. If you can't afford to get healthy, can you afford diabetes medications, high blood pressure meds, open heart surgery, depression meds, and more (the lists goes on)? If you don't try to get healthy, you set yourself up for dealing with—and paying for—all of the health problems that result from an unhealthy lifestyle. By investing in yourself now, you may avoid the high costs of an unhealthy lifestyle. Try this: If you're convinced that you *really* can't afford that gym membership, save all of your receipts from eating out for a couple of weeks. At the end of that time, see how

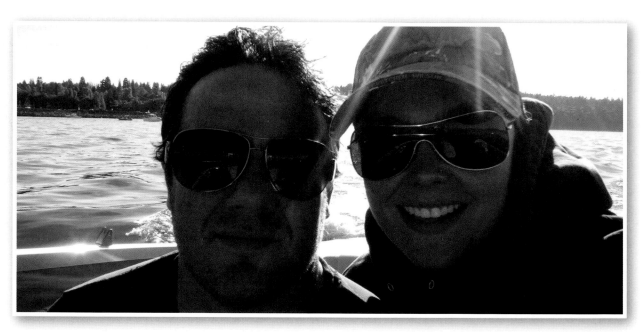

Boating on the Sound

much money you spent eating junk. I am willing to venture that more than likely you *can* afford a gym membership.

I won't lie: Eating healthy food can be a little costly, but as your lifestyle habits improve, you will find that you will have more money to use for the right things. For example, I didn't realize how much money I used to spend on alcohol. When I stopped drinking, it freed up a good amount of cash. If you are truly committed to a lifestyle change, take a look at your expenses. More than likely you have some habits that are costing you money right now that you don't even think about. Use the money you save from giving up these bad habits to supplement your new, healthy ones.

Question 3: Do you use a personal trainer, and what if I can't afford one?

I have an excellent trainer, and to me he is worth every cent that I pay him. He uses cutting-edge techniques to help me achieve my goals. I pay him, so I am more likely not to miss a workout (which is a good incentive for me). We have a great relationship, and he is not afraid to call me up and ask how things are going or where I have been if I have missed a workout for any reason. A trainer should help motivate you to push yourself beyond what you would do on your own, as well as educate you. Be wary of the trainer who always does the exact same routine or who you notice uses the same workout for every person. You are paying for a service and should expect to get results. Your trainer should customize your workout. If he or she is unwilling to, shop around. There are some excellent trainers out there that you deserve to use.

If you can't afford a trainer, don't worry about it. When you first started your job, did you know everything there was to know? I doubt it, but as you went to work everyday, you learned by doing, watching others, and asking questions. After a while, you probably became pretty proficient. Working out is similar to your first day on the job. First, show up and get acquainted with your surroundings. Find out where the equipment is, what it is, and how it works. Don't be afraid to ask questions. As intimidating as more seasoned people look working out, most are very willing to help out a beginner. Also, most gyms offer an orientation, so use it. Take advantage of all the classes and services that your particular gym offers. If they offer free classes, such as a spinning class, sign up for it and get going that way.

Question 4: What is the most difficult part of losing weight?

To be honest, losing weight was easy for me. Keeping it off has been the hardest part. Just like everyone else, I have days when I don't really want to work out and would love to stuff my face. Nowadays—as opposed to when I was at my biggest—I think about the consequences, as well as how I will feel if I do get off track. As I have said over and over, the only way to maintain weight loss is to continue to do the things that you did to lose it in the first place. There are temptations around every corner, and I have to have a battle plan ready at all times in order to be successful in maintaining my weight loss.

Question 5: I am worried about having saggy skin if I lose weight. Did you have that problem?

No, I didn't. I think that loose skin is more of a genetic thing, and it may be related to the general elasticity of your skin. There is no way to tell whether you will have it or not. If you are obese, there is a better chance than not that you will have some excess skin when you reach your lower weight, particularly if you've been overweight for longer than I was. That said, don't let a little, or even a lot, of excess skin be the reason you choose not to work out. Try to lose some fat weight. Consider the alternative: Carrying around excess fat is definitely not a better option.

This question always amuses me, because it shows me that the person is really looking for an excuse not to lose weight. I have yet to meet the person who says he or she is disappointed by losing weight because of getting saggy skin. If you are afraid of this, lose the weight first, and then worry about it. If you do have extra skin after weight loss, tuck it in.

If you decide to have surgery to remove it, be prepared for some serious recovery time. My wife had a complete beltectomy, which is a procedure in which the surgeon makes an incision all the way around the bikini line, as well as from mid chest down the middle of the body. After the incision, he or she cuts off the excess skin and then pulls the rest tight, stitches it up, and lets the healing process begin. It is major surgery, so my description is very inadequate. The recovery is actually a long and painful process; however, Suzy is glad she did it. There are definitely scars from the surgery, and I can not stress enough how vital it is to choose a reputable surgeon with many successful operations under his or her belt. If you choose this option, use the best surgeon you can find.

Question 6: I cheated and had laparoscopic (minimally invasive) gastric bypass surgery. How do I maintain my loss?

First of all, surgery is not cheating. It is a physically grueling experience, and it takes just as much effort to achieve results with it as a traditional diet. If surgery is your only option, I'm glad you took it. Once the surgery is over, you have to do the same things everyone else does: exercise and get proper nutrition. Post-surgery, people who choose not to adhere to their new lifestyle plan can gain the weight back as easily as anyone who was losing or maintaining weight on a more traditional diet and then stopped following it. In essence, to maintain your weight loss, you still have to maintain your healthy lifestyle just like anyone else.

Question 7: If you had to do it all over again, would you?

Absolutely! I can't thank *The Biggest Loser* enough for the changes that have occurred in my life as a direct result of being on the show. I have to believe that had I not been on, I would have maintained my unhealthy lifestyle and, more likely than not, would have suffered my first heart attack by now. Honestly, I have a new lease on life and truly appreciate all that I have been given. Not only do I have my beautiful bride, Suzy, and my little son, Rex, but I also have the confidence to overcome any obstacle that life throws in my way.

I know that all I dream of achieving can be done by setting my mind on it and then taking action. What's more, I am able to reach and help thousands of people through this experience and have found a career that

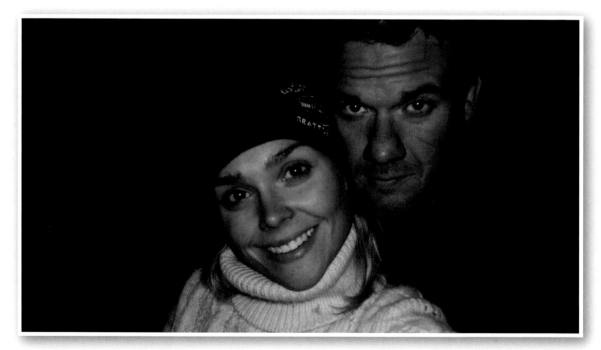

Late night on Manhattan Beach, California

suits me. All of these new things in my life could not have happened except by the grace of God, and I am forever a changed man. I will always have to keep a keen eye on my weight, but by changing my thinking, as well as my habits, it has become much easier to do and is more naturally just a part of my life.

Some Parting Thoughts

I would like to share one last personal story with you. When I left the Ranch, I decided to return to the University of Iowa to gain some closure on that part of my past.

I called Coach Gable and asked if I could come by to talk with him for a few minutes. It was time to explain what had happened during my time as a member of his team, apologize for not fulfilling my obligations, and thank him for having given me the opportunity to be a Hawkeye wrestler.

Coach Gable met me at his office in Carver Hawkeye Arena. It was my intention to just sit down and say "Thanks" and "I'm sorry," but as I began to speak, he said, "Hoover, I want to talk to you." I instantly began to sweat. Let me explain; from the time I began wrestling for him, Coach

Gable intimidated me. Every time he ever talked to me, I broke out in a cold sweat—not because of fear, but rather from being in the presence of greatness and excellence. He has always lived by the principles that he instilled in his wrestlers: Intensity, dedication, determination, strength, and integrity are a few that come to mind. I have only met a handful of people that I felt exhibited the traits they teach and claim to live by.

To be around a man who exemplifies such traits was intimidating to me. I now strive for that type of excellence in my own life.

So I was sweating and trying to think about what was coming next. The conversation that followed has had a profound impact on my life.

Coach Gable said, "Hoover, when you were here, you were always telling me what you were going to do. You were going to get

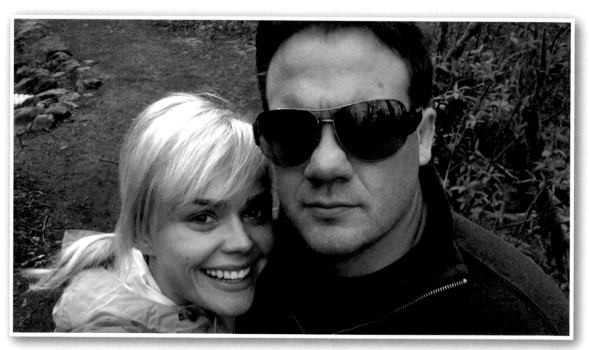

Suzy and me on the trail.

your grades up; you were going to get your weight under control; you were going to wrestle for me and become an all-American. Right after you got done telling me what you were going to do, you would tell me why you had to do it. You were ineligible, you hadn't worked out like you should, and what not.

"Hoov, you always told me what you were going to do and why, but you never told me what you were doing right then. See, I talk about the present as being the current. If your current isn't good, it's usually a result of your past not being too good. It's tough for things to go smoothly if you haven't had a good past or haven't taken care of the things that have happened in the past. The thing about your current not being good is that it makes it tough for your future to be good. If you're always worrying about the past or talking about what you are going to do in the future, you can't be taking care of your current. How's your current?"

It took me a while to digest the whole conversation, but I was instantly changed. I realized that I had definitely been either living in the past or in the future for quite some time and that in order for me to enjoy the life I desired, I needed to learn how to instead live in the present, or current. I understood that it didn't really matter what I had done in the past or what I was going to do in the future if I wasn't taking care of today. The only thing I have any control over is what is going on at this moment. By taking steps in my current every single day, I can achieve my goals for the future.

I don't have many bad days anymore, not because things never get tough for me, but rather because in the back of my mind I hold the question Coach Gable asked me that day in his office not so long ago. "Hoover, how's your current?"

We all need to stop wasting time trying to change things in the past that we can't change and worrying about things in the future that may or may not happen. Start living your new life today and pose this question to yourself: How *is* my current?

I can only hope that hearing my story has inspired you to take control of your weight and your health and will help you change your life for the better, too. Learn from my mistakes, change your habits, and do so now—before it's too late. I promise that you won't be sorry that you did. It's the only time in your life that being the biggest loser means that you're the biggest winner!

Suggested Reading

Alexander, Devin, et al. *The Biggest Loser Cookbook: More Than 125 Healthy, Delicious Recipes Adapted from NBC's Hit Show*. New York: Rodale Books, 2006.

Colberg, Sheri R. *The 7 Step Diabetes Fitness Plan: Living Well and Being Fit with Diabetes, No Matter Your Weight*. New York: Marlowe & Company, 2006.

Morley, John E., and Sheri R. Colberg. *The Science of Staying Young*. New York: McGraw-Hill, 2007.

Stein, Richard. *Outliving Heart Disease: The 10 New Rules for Prevention and Treatment*. New York: Newmarket Press, 2006.

The Biggest Loser Experts and Cast. *The Biggest Loser: The Weight Loss Program to Transform Your Body, Health, and Life*. New York: Rodale Books, 2005.

The Biggest Loser Experts and Cast. *The Biggest Loser Calorie Counter: The Quick and Easy Guide to Thousands of Foods from Grocery Stores and Popular Restaurants*. New York: Rodale Books, 2006.

The Biggest Loser Experts and Cast, and Maggie Greenwood-Robinson. *The Biggest Loser Fitness Program: Fast, Safe, and Effective Workouts to Target and Tone Your Trouble Spots*. New York: Rodale Books, 2007.

Selected References by Chapter

Chapter 1

Geier, A. B., Schwartz, M. B., Brownell, K. D. "'Before and after' diet advertisements escalate weight stigma." *Eating and Weight Disorders*. 2003, 8(4): 282–8.

The Biggest Loser Club Web site. Accessed on April 17, 2008. www.nbc.com/The_Biggest_Loser/club

Chapter 2

Carr, D., Friedman, M. A. "Is obesity stigmatizing? Body weight, perceived discrimination, and psychological well-being in the United States." *Journal of Health and Social Behavior*. 2005, 46(3): 244–59.

Oppliger, R. A., Steen, S. A., Scott, J. R. "Weight loss practices of college wrestlers." *International Journal of Sport Nutrition and Exercise Metabolism*. 2003, 13(1): 29–46.

Oppliger, R. A., Utter, A. C., Scott, J. R., Dick, R. W., Klossner, D. "NCAA rule change improves weight loss among national championship wrestlers." *Medicine and Science in Sports and Exercise.* 2006, 38(5): 963–70.

Schwartz, M. B., Chambliss, H. O., Brownell, K. D., Blair, S. N., Billington, C. "Weight bias among health professionals specializing in obesity." *Obesity Research.* 2003, 11(9): 1033–9.

Schwartz M. B., Vartanian L. R., Nosek B. A., Brownell K. D. "The influence of one's own body weight on implicit and explicit anti-fat bias." *Obesity.* 2006; 14(3): 440–7.

Stephan, Y., Bilard, J. "Repercussions of transition out of elite sport on body image." *Perceptual and Motor Skills.* 2003, 96(1): 95–104.

Ungerleider, S. "Olympic athletes' transition from sport to workplace." *Perceptual and Motor Skills.* 1997, 84(3 Pt 2): 1287–95.

Chapter 3

Dansinger, M. L., Gleason, J. A., Griffith, J. L., Selker, H. P., Schaefer, E. J. "Comparison of the Atkins, Ornish, Weight Watchers, and Zone diets for weight loss and heart disease risk reduction: a randomized trial." *Journal of the American Medical Association.* 2005, 293(1): 43–53.

Fleming, R. M. "The effect of high-, moderate-, and low-fat diets on weight loss and cardiovascular disease risk factors." *Preventive Cardiology.* 2002, 5(3): 110–8.

Gardner, C. D., Kiazand, A., Alhassan, S., Kim, S., Stafford, R. S., Balise, R. R., Kraemer, H. C., King, A. C. "Comparison of the Atkins, Zone, Ornish, and LEARN diets for change in weight and related risk factors among overweight premenopausal women: the A TO Z Weight Loss Study: a randomized trial." *Journal of the American Medical Association.* 2007, 297(9): 969–77.

Kruger, J., Blanck, H. M., Gillespie, C. "Dietary and physical activity behaviors among adults successful at weight loss maintenance." *International Journal of Behavioral Nutrition and Physical Activity*. 2006, 3: 17.

McAuley, K. A., Hopkins, C. M., Smith, K. J., McLay, R. T., Williams, S. M., Taylor, R. W., Mann, J. I. "Comparison of high-fat and high-protein diets with a high-carbohydrate diet in insulin-resistant obese women." *Diabetologia*. 2005, 48(1): 8–16.

Phelan, S., Wyatt, H. R., Hill, J. O., Wing, R. R. "Are the eating and exercise habits of successful weight losers changing?" *Obesity*. 2006, 14(4): 710–6.

Phelan, S., Wyatt, H., Nassery, S., Dibello, J., Fava, J. L., Hill, J. O., Wing, R. R. "Three-year weight change in successful weight losers who lost weight on a low-carbohydrate diet." *Obesity*. 2007, 15(10): 2470–7.

Pi-Sunyer, F. X., Aronne, L. J., Heshmati, H. M., Devin, J., Rosenstock, J.; RIO-North America Study Group. "Effect of rimonabant, a cannabinoid-1 receptor blocker, on weight and cardiometabolic risk factors in overweight or obese patients: RIO-North America: a randomized controlled trial." *Journal of the American Medical Association*. 2006, 295(7): 761–75.

Raynor, H. A., Jeffery, R. W., Phelan, S., Hill, J. O., Wing, R. R. "Amount of food group variety consumed in the diet and long-term weight loss maintenance." *Obesity Research*. 2005, 13(5): 883–90.

Shick, S. M., Wing, R. R., Klem, M. L., McGuire, M. T., Hill, J. O., Seagle, H. "Persons successful at long-term weight loss and maintenance continue to consume a low-energy, low-fat diet." *Journal of the American Dietetics Association*. 1998, 98(4): 408–13.

Chapter 4

Cosca, D. D., Navazio, F. "Common problems in endurance athletes." *American Family Physician*. 2007, 76(2): 237–44.

Gibala, M. J., Little, J. P., van Essen, M., Wilkin, G. P., Burgomaster, K. A., Safdar, A., Raha, S., Tarnopolsky, M. A. "Short-term sprint interval versus traditional endurance training: similar initial adaptations in human skeletal muscle and exercise performance." *Journal of Physiology*. 2006, 575(Pt 3): 901–11.

Hamilton, M. T., Hamilton, D. G., Zderic, T. W. "Role of low energy expenditure and sitting in obesity, metabolic syndrome, type 2 diabetes, and cardiovascular disease." *Diabetes*. 2007, 56(11): 2655–67.

Haskell, W. L., Lee, I. M., Pate, R. R., Powell, K. E., Blair, S. N., Franklin, B. A., Macera, C. A., Heath, G. W., Thompson, P. D., Bauman, A. "Physical activity and public health: updated recommendation for adults from the American College of Sports Medicine and the American Heart Association." *Medicine and Science in Sports and Exercise*. 2007, 39(8): 1423–34.

Kruger, J., Blanck, H. M., Gillespie, C. "Dietary and physical activity behaviors among adults successful at weight loss maintenance." *International Journal of Behavioral Nutrition and Physical Activity*. 2006, 3: 17.

Leser, M. S., Yanovski, S. Z., Yanovski, J. A. "A low-fat intake and greater activity level are associated with lower weight regain 3 years after completing a very-low-calorie diet." *Journal of the American Dietetics Association*. 2002, 102(9): 1252–6.

Levine, J. A., Schleusner, S. J., Jensen, M. D. "Energy expenditure of nonexercise activity." *American Journal of Clinical Nutrition*. 2000, 72(6): 1451–4.

Nelson, M. E., Rejeski, W. J., Blair, S. N., Duncan, P. W., Judge, J. O., King, A. C., Macera, C. A., Castaneda-Sceppa, C. "Physical activity and public health in older adults:

recommendation from the American College of Sports Medicine and the American Heart Association." *Medicine and Science in Sports and Exercise.* 2007, 39(8): 1435–45.

Stevens, J., Cai, J., Evenson, K. R., Thomas, R. "Fitness and fatness as predictors of mortality from all causes and from cardiovascular disease in men and women in the lipid research clinics study." *American Journal of Epidemiology.* 2002, 156(9): 832–41.

Vogels, N., Westerterp-Plantenga, M. S. "Successful long-term weight maintenance: a 2-year follow-up." *Obesity.* 2007, 15(5): 1258–66.

Zainuddin, Z., Newton, M., Sacco, P., Nosaka, K. "Effects of massage on delayed-onset muscle soreness, swelling, and recovery of muscle function." *Journal of Athletic Training.* 2005, 40(3): 174–80.

Chapter 5

Campbell, W. K., Foster, C. A., Finkel, E. J. "Does self-love lead to love for others? A story of narcissistic game playing." *Journal of Personality and Social Psychology.* 2002, 83(2): 340–54.

Hanson, K. L., Sobal, J., Frongillo, E. A. "Gender and marital status clarify associations between food insecurity and body weight." *Journal of Nutrition.* 2007, 137(6): 1460–5.

Marigold, D. C., Holmes, J. G., Ross, M. "More than words: reframing compliments from romantic partners fosters security in low self-esteem individuals." *Journal of Personality and Social Psychology.* 2007, 92(2): 232–48

Sobal, J., Nicolopoulos, V., Lee, J. "Attitudes about overweight and dating among secondary school students." *International Journal of Obesity and Related Metabolic Disorders.* 1995, 19(6): 376–81.

Chapter 6

Haskell, C. F., Kennedy, D. O., Wesnes, K. A., Scholey, A. B. "Cognitive and mood improvements of caffeine in habitual consumers and habitual non-consumers of caffeine." *Psychopharmacology*. 2005, 179(4): 813–25.

Khan, S., Evans, A. A., Hughes, S., Smith, M. E. "Beta-endorphin decreases fatigue and increases glucose uptake independently in normal and dystrophic mice." *Muscle and Nerve*. 2005, 31(4): 481–6.

Marigold, D. C., Holmes, J. G., Ross, M. "More than words: reframing compliments from romantic partners fosters security in low self-esteem individuals." *Journal of Personality and Social Psychology*. 2007, 92(2): 232–48

Pasman, W. J., Blokdijk, V. M., Bertina, F. M., Hopman, W. P., Hendriks, H. F. "Effect of two breakfasts, different in carbohydrate composition, on hunger and satiety and mood in healthy men." *International Journal of Obesity and Related Metabolic Disorders*. 2003, 27(6): 663–8.

Chapter 7

Anderson, J. W., Conley, S. B., Nicholas, A. S. "One hundred pound weight losses with an intensive behavioral program: changes in risk factors in 118 patients with long-term follow-up." *American Journal of Clinical Nutrition*. 2007, 86(2): 301–7.

Bellisle, F., Dalix, A. M., De Assis, M. A., Kupek, E., Gerwig, U., Slama, G., Oppert, J. M. "Motivational effects of 12-week moderately restrictive diets with or without special attention to the Glycaemic Index of foods." *British Journal of Nutrition*. 2007, 97(4): 790–8.

National Heart, Lung, and Blood Institute: Key Recommendations from the Expert Panel on the Identification, Evaluation, and Treatment of Overweight and Obesity in Adults. Accessed on April 18, 2008, www.nhlbi.nih.gov/guidelines/obesity/ob_gdlns.htm/

Nothwehr, F., Yang, J. "Goal setting frequency and the use of behavioral strategies related to diet and physical activity." *Health Education Research*. 2007, 22(4): 532–8.

Sabinsky, M. S., Toft, U., Raben, A., Holm, L. "Overweight men's motivations and perceived barriers towards weight loss." *European Journal of Clinical Nutrition*. 2007, 61(4): 526–31.

Chapter 8

Field, A. E., Austin, S. B., Taylor, C. B., Malspeis, S., Rosner, B., Rockett, H. R., Gillman, M. W., Colditz, G. A. "Relation between dieting and weight change among preadolescents and adolescents." *Pediatrics*. 2003, 112(4): 900–6.

Leser, M. S., Yanovski, S. Z., Yanovski, J. A. "A low-fat intake and greater activity level are associated with lower weight regain 3 years after completing a very-low-calorie diet." *Journal of the American Dietetics Association*. 2002, 102(9): 1252–6.

Oddy, W. H., Li, J., Landsborough, L., Kendall, G. E., Henderson, S., Downie, J. "The association of maternal overweight and obesity with breastfeeding duration." *Journal of Pediatrics*. 2006, 149(2): 185–91.

Raynor, H. A., Jeffery, R. W., Phelan, S., Hill, J. O., Wing, R. R. "Amount of food group variety consumed in the diet and long-term weight loss maintenance." *Obesity Research*. 2005, 13(5): 883–90.

Rodearmel, S. J., Wyatt, H. R., Stroebele, N., Smith, S. M., Ogden, L. G., Hill, J. O. "Small changes in dietary sugar and physical activity as an approach to preventing excessive weight gain: the America on the Move family study." *Pediatrics*. 2007, 120(4): e869–79.

Vogels, N., Westerterp-Plantenga, M. S. "Successful long-term weight maintenance: a 2-year follow-up." *Obesity*. 2007, 15(5): 1258–66.

Acknowledgments

First and foremost, we owe our thanks to our families for standing by us (or, more accurately, getting by without us) while we worked on this book. Matt is forever grateful for the loving support he received from his wife, Suzy, while Dr. Sheri again thanks her husband, Ray Ochs, and her three sons for being so understanding of the time that goes into creating a book that is worthy of being published.

Next, we appreciate the support of all the crew at Skyhorse Publishing, including our editor, Abigail Gehring, and many other hard-working individuals behind the scenes at this publishing house. Finally, we also owe many thanks to our literary agent, Linda Konner, for her belief in this book and our ability to get it written in time. She is a true champion in the cause for weight control and healthy living.

About the Authors

Matt Hoover was the grand prize winner of NBC's *The Biggest Loser 2*. A legend back in his hometown of Belle Plaine, Iowa, he was a member of four NCAA wrestling championship teams at the University of Iowa. In high school, Matt was a two-time Iowa state wrestling champion and was thrice named a high school all-American athlete. Awarded a scholarship to the top college wrestling program in the nation at the University of Iowa, he was later torn from his Olympic dreams by an injury, leaving his competitive dreams unfilled. After his wrestling career ended, he developed severe eating and drinking problems that caused his weight to balloon up to 340 pounds in just a few years. Near the height of his weight gain and the nadir of his life, he was cast to be on the NBC show *The Biggest Loser 2* early in 2005. He arrived at the Biggest Loser Ranch in March of 2005 weighing 339 pounds, but ended up winning the show's grand prize by losing 157 pounds in just nine months. He weighed in at only 182 pounds at the final weigh-in—thus accomplishing a remarkable 46.31 percent overall weight loss (close to half his body weight).

Matt Hoover currently resides with his wife, Suzy Preston Hoover, near Seattle, Washington. He works as a motivational speaker, traveling around the country, and he also coaches individuals on exercise training regimens and works with many others to help them achieve their weight loss goals. He and his wife welcomed their first child, Rex, in the summer of 2007.

Sheri R. Colberg, PhD, is an exercise physiologist and professor of exercise science at Old Dominion University in Norfolk, Virginia, as well as the executive director of the Lifelong Exercise Institute (LEI, accessible at www.lifelongexercise.com). Having earned a PhD from the University of California, Berkeley, she specializes in research on exercise, particularly related to obesity, diabetes control, lifestyle improvements, and prevention of chronic health problems. She has also authored more than 150 research and educational articles on exercise, nutrition, weight loss, diabetes, and aging (many accessible at www.shericolberg.com), as well as six books: *The Diabetic Athlete, Diabetes-Free Kids, The 7 Step Diabetes Fitness Plan, 50 Secrets of the Longest Living People with Diabetes, The Science of Staying Young,* and *The Diabetic Athlete's Handbook.* A person living long and well with type 1 diabetes since the age of four, she practices what she preaches when it comes to living a healthy lifestyle and exercising daily. A resident of Virginia Beach, Virginia, with her husband and their three sons, she is an avid recreational exerciser who enjoys swimming, biking, walking, tennis, weight training, hiking, and yard work, as well as staying active with her boys.

ML   10/08